HATCHING

HATCHING

*Experiments in Motherhood
and Technology*

Jenni Quilter

RIVERHEAD BOOKS · NEW YORK · 2022

RIVERHEAD BOOKS
An imprint of Penguin Random House LLC
penguinrandomhouse.com

Copyright © 2022 by Jennifer Quilter

Grateful acknowledgment is made for permission to reprint lines from
"A Wave" by John Ashbery. Copyright © 1981, 1982, 1983, 1984 by John Ashbery.
Reprinted by permission of Georges Borchardt, Inc.,
on behalf of the author. All rights reserved.

Library of Congress Control Number: 2022001714

ISBN 9780735213203 (hardcover)
ISBN 9780735213227 (ebook)

Printed in the United States of America
1st Printing

BOOK DESIGN BY LUCIA BERNARD

For Stephanie

. . .

Contents

HATCHING

1

· · ·

GRAFT

Occasionally there are books that you encounter like arrows: they arrive with velocity and a distinct *whump*. Naomi Mitchison's *Memoirs of a Spacewoman* was like that for me. It was published in 1962, and I picked it up around 2017. It's not widely known. The book collects the "expedition notes" of a spacewoman called Mary and her visits to various planets, and it is the ventriloquized voice of the future, a way for Mitchison to imagine the fantasies and freedoms she thought the future might afford a woman like her.

It's not that Mitchison hadn't already carved out for herself an extraordinarily rich and varied life. By the time *Memoirs* came out, she was sixty-five years old and living in Scotland. She had given birth to seven children, traveled extensively, and openly talked about her open marriage (her only regret, she said on her ninetieth birthday, were all the men with whom she didn't sleep). Then there were the political appointments, and numerous societies, commissions, and councils, many of them revolving around socialism, birth control, and Scottish economic development. She wrote, by her own account, compulsively, and though *Memoirs of a Spacewoman* was her first science-fiction novel, she had already published dozens of books by then: mostly novels, but also travel writing and autobiography. She would go on to write more than ninety books by her death, in 1999, at 101.

Mitchison was very matter-of-fact about all this in her memoirs, and Mary, the narrator, is similarly prosaic: in the novel, the extraordinary isn't ordinary, but it shouldn't be considered any kind of rare or bizarre exception; for all we know, there could be hundreds of Marys in space, and we just happen to be reading about this one.

Mary has six children. Four of the children are human, and two are alien. One child, Ariel, is a tentacle-like creature with whom Mary communicates through number theory (the tentacle can tap out number sequences on her leg). Another, Viola, is described as half-human, half-Martian. Mary conceives a few of these children back on Earth, and a few in space. Some, but not all, have biological fathers. Mary does not raise all of them together. In this new world, her age has nothing to do with her reproductive clock. Because time moves more slowly away from Earth, and because she embarks on a number of space missions to different worlds and solar systems, each time Mary returns to Earth she returns to a different world: there is no one who ages contiguously with her, no lover, no family, not even her own children, who are infants when she embarks on one trip, then teenagers when she returns—and she has only aged a year. The work of child-rearing, all the dinners and washing and endless negotiations, can be excised in one hyperspace leap. Mary mentions feeling guilty only once.

For anyone who has felt the queasiness of pregnancy, the sudden conviction that your body is not your own, the inner roiling and the splitting open, the endless days and nights of cleaning and feeding,

Mitchison's freedoms are fascinating. For anyone who has not fallen pregnant or raised a child, but who has been caught between the fearing and the yearning, Mitchison's recasting of the obligations of parenthood is also irresistible. Mary has a biologist's eye in her attention to cause and effect, and is obviously interested in how our physiological structure directs our cognitive and moral frameworks. Her tone is professional, even impassive: she sees no disconnect between scientific exploration and reproduction, and is not surprised that her expeditions involve physiological experiments of more than one kind. Her pregnancies defamiliarize two discourses—one of scientific knowledge, the other of motherhood—at the same time. Her acts of conceiving are not something you balance with work: it *is* the work. This conceptual reorganization is akin to a shift from ptolemaic to heliocentric conceptions of the universe. The baby is no longer the thing around which everything revolves. Rather, it's the woman's body, and her decision to experiment with it. How one *feels*—cramps, blood, cell growth and death, hormone swings—is a site of analysis rather than a vaguely taboo topic.

The first time I read *Memoirs of a Spacewoman*, I felt relief so strongly that it registered as a kind of digestive ache. Here was a woman who had thought about birth in terms I instinctively understood but rarely recognized in the world around me.

Mitchison grew up in Oxford, England, the daughter of a scientist, and was educated at the well-regarded Dragon School, the only girl in a classroom of boys. She was regularly allowed into her father's laboratory. With her brother, J. B. S. Haldane, she carried out a number of experiments exploring Mendelian inheritance patterns in guinea pigs. These were all good augurs for her intellectual independence, but when she turned fourteen, her parents decided to homeschool her rather than send her away to boarding school as they did with her brother. Although she later studied at the University of Oxford, she was a "day student," enrolled in a women's college that had a different course of instruction than her brother's college, barely a mile away. Mitchison knew what she was missing out on because her brother allowed her to pal around with his friends in his college rooms. It was Haldane, not Mitchison, who published their early genetic experiments with guinea pigs, and it was her brother who, in 1924, published a small pamphlet titled *Daedalus; or, Science and the Future*, which described a future in which children would be grown in artificial wombs. Although Mitchison had been taught the pleasures of intellectual independence, no one actually expected her to use her mind to make a living. Education was an enrichment rather than a necessity. By her own account, she married young in order to achieve freedom from her family.

As a young woman, I had more freedom than Mitchison did. I was able to attend school as a teenager. I left my country—Aotearoa, New Zealand—to study and later teach at Oxford University, where I regularly cycled the road north from town, past Mitchison's family house. I did not have to marry to escape anything. My economic independence was precarious, and completely necessary. To make ends meet as a graduate student, I tutored at multiple colleges throughout the town; by the time I left, I had lived at five colleges, and taught in at least seven. I knew the strange eddies of thinking that were created when academics of different stripes dined with each other, night after night. It was not a surprise to me that a speculative fascination with babies in bottles ran like a current through J. B. S. Haldane's and Mitchison's social set: one of Haldane's friends at Oxford, who became close to Mitchison too, was the writer Aldous Huxley. Huxley went on to write probably the most famous novelistic exploration of ectogenesis (the development of embryos in artificial conditions outside the uterus) in *Brave New World*, which memorably features a vast room filled with row upon row of babies in bottles. Aldous's brother, Julian Huxley, also wrote speculative science fiction, including a short story, "The Tissue-Culture King," which focused on assembly-line biology. Mitchison's brother, Haldane, did the same: his pamphlet *Daedalus* begins as an attempt to predict the future, and quietly ends up as a short story narrated as history: it was in 1951, he wrote (in 1924), that Dupont and Schwartz produced the first ectogenetic child. By 1968, Haldane "reported," France was producing 60,000 children annually. It wasn't just the Huxleys and Haldane who were interested in ectogenesis: their friends and colleagues Vera Brittain and J. D. Bernal wrote about it too.

These writers published their work on artificial wombs in the 1920s and '30s, but Mitchison didn't publish *Memoirs of a Spacewoman* until 1962. When it came out, Huxley was living in Los Angeles, suffering from laryngeal cancer. He would die a year later. Mitchison's brother, fed up with English political life, had also emigrated, to India, in 1956. Huxley, Haldane, and Mitchison, who had spent so much of their youth together in Oxford, were each now living on what were virtually different planets. It's quite possible that neither man read *Memoirs*: Haldane would die only a year after Huxley. I have found no mention in their correspondence that they received the novel. If they didn't—well, it saddens me. They supported Mitchison, and I think they would've been fascinated by how she refigured their own rewirings of reproduction and sexuality.

In *Brave New World*, women have been "liberated" from the burden of child rearing and are free to have sex with whomever they please. The novel is obviously dystopian, partly because sexuality (without procreation) is understood as an anti-cultural force, as a reason why people are shallow and incurious: all pleasure, no purpose. This is not a world that is interested in depth: the artificial womb has collapsed interior space. J. B. S. Haldane's account of ectogenesis is more positive, but still rather ominous in that he focuses, like Huxley, on change writ large, on percentages and years. The implications are consequential, but kept at arm's length. But Mitchison's vision is fundamentally more optimistic. She keeps her focus on the individual: her novel is not about glass bottles, kept at a remove, but about what it is like to *be* the bottle, to be the site of the experiment. The dominant mode is exploration rather than escape. She isn't interested in a collapsing world as much as an expanding one.

Mitchison lived long enough to see the growth of new reproductive technologies as an industry, for biologically female women to become the bottle on *terra firma*. For decades now, people have chosen to undergo in vitro fertilization, more commonly known as IVF. We can fall pregnant without sperm entering the cervix; fall pregnant with eggs that have been harvested from our own bodies years before; develop in our uterus or someone else's a child that isn't genetically ours. Reproductive time travel has become a standard news item in the late twentieth and early twenty-first century: twins born to a sixty-seven-year-old woman, or a grandmother acting as a surrogate for her own daughter, carrying and giving birth to her grandson. With each announcement, newspapers reliably trot out a *Brave New World* analogy or pun. What might have been if Mitchison's novel, rather than Huxley's, was our automatic cultural touchstone for thinking about experiments in childbearing? What anchoring effect might her speculative fiction have had on our own sense of reproductive possibility?

In *Memoirs of a Spacewoman*, Mary's job is to work as an empath, tasked with communicating with alien life forms. As she notes on more than one occasion, "Communication science is so essentially womanly. It fits one's basic sex patterns." When I first read the novel, the claim irked me. I was reading it in my thirties, when my gender, which had never felt like much of a constraint, started to tighten, like suddenly snug pants. I defensively bristled at categorizations. Why, I thought, would you create gendered expectations in your fiction if you spent most of your life resisting their limitations? Wouldn't Mitchison be more interested in the *dissolution* of gender than in its confirmation?

But focusing on a woman's empathy allowed Mitchison to explore her own ambivalences about the concept. More than once, Mary starts to experience a disintegration of self because she is so empathetic. The most straightforward example of this is in her first expedition, which involves a species "like a five-armed starfish," which ranges in size from a few centimeters to a meter across. Trying to communicate with these creatures, Mary acknowledges "how much we are ourselves constructed bi-laterally on either-or principles.... One is so used to a two-sided brain, two eyes, two ears, and so on that one takes the whole thing and all that stems from it for granted." After some time in the company of these alien starfish, Mary realizes she cannot think in binary terms or make either/or decisions. She begins to forget her name. Of encounters with other life-forms, she explains that communicators like her cannot "integrate" for too long, because their personality will degrade, even disintegrate. She says this so matter-of-factly that it takes a moment to register that this disintegration is sped up by her pregnancies—spelling out implications for motherhood that, in popular culture, we tend to dance around. Empathy has a cost. The novel, it turns out, is also a series of meditations on subsuming yourself to another creature.

None of this was technically news to me about the costs of becoming a parent. I was ambivalent about becoming a mother because I could see how difficult it would be to balance the work of focusing on a child with focusing on a career. I could see how exhausted my friends with children were. But the harassed-looking parent is such a common trope that it is easy to accept—and rationalize—without thinking too deeply about the costs that parenthood exacts. If one speaks of the pain, one is preternaturally quick to also speak of the love and joy that children bring. In Mitchison's novel, that cost is starkly rendered. Mary nearly dies. She loses relationships. She loses a child. None of it is recuperable or absorbable, and that's not how Mitchison would rationalize it. She is placing a woman's reproductive ability at the center of a cosmology of knowledge and exploration, and is willing to understand it as a risk taken for knowledge, rather than some kind of biological inevitability or "fact of life."

In part, this book tries to take Mitchison's sense of risk-for-knowledge just as seriously, focusing on how it plays out on Earth in real time rather than as speculative science fiction. The technology of IVF was developed because thousands upon thousands of un-named women chose to experiment with their bodies, knowing how unlikely it was that they would become pregnant. Right now, the odds of a successful pregnancy through IVF (depending on maternal age) hover at around 35 percent. In the early 1980s, it was approximately 5 percent. The technology has also developed within a much longer medical tradition of experimenting on women *without* requiring their clear and informed consent. It is hard to know whether one is a guinea pig or a moral pioneer or both when it comes to new reproductive technologies.

The revolutionary potential Mitchison imagined—her disaggregation of the time of the body from the time of parenting, monogamy from motherhood—has barely been realized. IVF clinics unthinkingly, even compulsively, offer a heterosexual cisgender dream of a nuclear family. One could attempt to create a family structure that is not normative, but it can be so routinely mistaken for more traditional forms that any transgressive implications are quietly and constantly managed away. Within an IVF clinic, exploring "one's options" tends to be in the interests of structural repetition rather than of exploring new forms of kinship.

These options are also strictly defined by class and race. Experimental reproduction, in Mitchison's novel and in our world today, tends to be for white women who can afford it. This is not something Mitchison reflects on consciously in her novel; indeed, it's one of the book's blind spots. The money required to raise Mary's children is simply not mentioned, which appears to vanquish the question of class. Race is recast as cosmic biodiversity. She only has sex with male humans or aliens. The freedom given to the spacewoman is "simply" a function of space travel and science, rather than a named political belief. The epistemological shell game in this novel is that any feminism always turns out to be science.

As a white Pākehā woman who could also afford to experiment, I am interested in what and how I have been taught to desire when it comes to the question of reproduction. Why is it so difficult to become a spacewoman in one's own life? Mary is able to put her life on Earth to one side; it barely takes up six or so sentences in Mitchison's book. My interest is in what enmeshes us, drawing us back to forms of living we have little interest in replicating, yet nonetheless continue. These forms of learning are deep-rooted; if Mitchison casts herself forward in time, I move backward, charting the development of technologies for viewing and manipulating female-identified bodies from the sixteenth century onward, and noting how we have been taught to understand the reproductive potential of our bodies: what it means to conceive or *not* to conceive, to carry a fetus to term or abort one, to raise a child. We have been trained to understand the insides and outsides of our bodies in very particular ways, and how we visualize our bodies' limits determines our aim, what arc of ambition we might cast in our lives. So much of our sight has been delimited by shame about certain parts of the body and how they function. Only a select number of bodily transformations are celebrated; others are minimized, muted, dismissed as a side effect rather than an event with epistemological consequences. We are taught to dismiss or interpret signs in our bodies that could be valued very differently if we placed them inside other cosmologies of learning: a clinical diagnosis of infertility, for example, can be understood not just with a WebMD article, but in relation to a history of how the egg has been viewed and conceptualized. The consumerism of pregnancy—which seems mostly unavoidable, at least in the United States—is intimately tied to our sense of the domestic, when it need not be. There are other ways to structure a home.

I have thought of Mitchison many times in writing my own expedition notes, more than half a century later. I have wondered about the relationship between Naomi, the writer, and Mary, the spacewoman. They are related, and not identical: another kind of reproduction. To write about one's blood, one's milk—to record the effects of a body in time—creates a new corpus, a phantom body that has also grown and walked with me these past five years. She now leaves me, and goes to you.*

---

*Throughout this book, I write that women give birth to babies. This, as we know, isn't true: women who have transitioned to another gender identity can also give birth. Motherhood and fatherhood and parenthood can be one and the same, though this is obscured by the text's frequent association of cisgendered women with motherhood. Some of this is historical; most of the sources I discuss assume there are two genders assigned at birth that do not change. Where possible, I've tried to quietly point these assumptions out. I've also tried to make my own language more inclusive to a variety of expressions of gender. I do not want my account to efface the accounts of others. And yet so much of this book is also about being identified by others *as* a woman, and the swiftness of this categorization is, I think, a central part of my experience. To *not* show this risks a level of retroactive narrative contortion that ends up effacing the social forces at work here: our desire to gender is part and parcel of IVF's conservatism. There are also times when I come very close to aligning femininity with motherhood because various experiences of one category ended up teaching me something about the other. *This is only because it happened that way for me*: I am allergic to expectations that either category "should" perform in certain ways, and my interest is not in shoring up gender expectations as much as questioning them, with all my blind spots as a white, able-bodied, middle-class woman.

2

. . .

14.3

On the 28th of June, 2015, a nurse rang me up and told me—in a conversation that lasted less than thirty seconds—that at the age of thirty-five, I did not have the eggs I should have. In medical terms, this is called diminished ovarian reserve. Contrary to how I looked and felt, to statistical norms and inheritance patterns, one part of my body was aging faster than the rest. My cupboard was bare.

I had expected to begin stimulating my ovaries that day. In the morning, I went into the clinic for an ultrasound and blood work. They saw eight follicles in my ovaries, which are the casings that eggs grow in; it wasn't a huge number, but it wasn't terrible either. My blood work said something else: my FSH (follicle-stimulating hormone) level was very high for my age, which meant that the hormones I was planning to inject myself with probably wouldn't work; I wouldn't grow follicles *en masse* so that they could be retrieved two weeks later. My AMH (anti-Müllerian hormone) number was also too low, which indicated I had very few eggs left. These numbers were more appropriate for a woman in her forties, not her thirties.

When I asked to talk to the doctor, the nurse told me he would ring the next day. And then she hung up.

I had been lying on the couch when she rang and for a minute or two, I didn't move. I thought about the medicine in my bedroom, which had been delivered by FedEx in two large boxes the day before, and which I had laid out on a bookshelf: large packs of syringes and different gauge needles, vials and micro-fine injection pins, needle disposal containers, box after box of the different medicines. Some of it needed to be refrigerated, and I'd made room for it all: milk, pickles, Follistim. The medicine had cost approximately $8,000.

I had spent the previous two weeks preparing myself for the next two weeks. I had undergone an HSG (hysterosalpingography), which involved flushing iodinated water through my fallopian tubes and uterus and X-raying the glowing lines of liquid to check for blockages. I had watched videos of how to administer the two to four injections I'd need every day. I knew how to load a Follistim pen cartridge, how to set the dosage, how to pinch my stomach so there was a roll of flesh for the needle to enter. I had accepted the likely side effects, which included weight gain, bloating, cramping, mood swings, and headaches. I knew I wouldn't be able to do yoga, or cycle, or even swim. Twisting the torso can damage the swollen ovaries—each of which can grow to be between the size of a lemon and a grapefruit. Now none of that mattered.

I walked over to the table and my laptop, and typed my FSH and AMH numbers into Google. This was one of the first paragraphs I read, from the Reproductive Medicine Associates of Michigan: "Essentially, an elevated Day 3 FSH value indicates a very poor prognosis for conception through IVF and a high risk of pregnancy loss should the rare conception occur. Unfortunately, if you ever exhibit an elevated FSH value, having a normal value at a later time does not favorably change this prognosis. . . . At RMA, we have determined that an FSH value of 15 or higher predicts that IVF will be of no value in helping to achieve pregnancy. FSH values over 14.5 have produced only rare pregnancies in our program."

No value. My FSH was 14.3. (For most women my age, it is under 10.) The website went on to recommend egg donation, which is when you pay for another woman's eggs, which are then fertilized and transferred to your uterus. My genetic line would end with me.

Most health organizations define a woman's infertility as the inability to fall pregnant after a year of unprotected sexual intercourse with a man, but that wasn't the way I came to the word. When I was thirty-five, I decided to freeze my eggs; I wasn't in a relationship, and I wanted to make sure it would be possible to have a baby later. I had always been ambivalent about having children; someday, but not right now. I had not fantasized about babies, had not grown up with them, did not babysit them. In fact, up until that point I couldn't even remember holding a single baby in my life. I knew I must've held them, but I couldn't recall the actual experience: I had never sniffed their heads, or felt their tiny arms around my neck, and couldn't imagine staring at their faces or playing with their fingers. I had missed the boat, I thought, on craving motherhood.

But when I found out about my egg supply, I was devastated. I spent most of my days on the internet, reading about those hormone results. I was introduced to countless narratives, much like the one you're reading right now, all which recounted numbers, attempts, failures, successes. I didn't want to work, eat, or see friends. The solidity of things had changed. What had once been bulwarks in my world—solitude, work, exhilaration—hollowed out, dissolved, and I was left with dust in my mouth. I found myself caring very little about the future. Why, if I had been so ambivalent, had I stumbled upon such a vast plain of grief? Did I not know myself? I did not buy the thought that this panic was "simply" my biological clock; my egg supply had probably been low for some time, and I hadn't even known. Nor did I want to accept that it was just the usual career-gal, have-it-all panic that newspaper columnists love to sermonize about, disapproving of the desire to fit, Tetris-like, the blocks of a relationship and a career and a baby into one life. This didn't feel like an existential hissy fit. At least, I hoped not.

Years later, writing this down, I am surprised by how matter-of-fact I can now be. At the time, I was undone.

I had underestimated the structural logic of motherhood. When I was in my twenties, I read about image schemas, which were a fancy way of naming recurring structures in our cognitive processes which establish patterns of understanding and reasoning. According to this theory, our bodily experiences as babies direct our later linguistic experiences and expressions: our most basic spatial patterns (in/out, up/down, etc.) structure figurative language and abstract reasoning. For example, we metaphorically project the spatial direction "out" without thinking twice into more-conceptual sentences like "Tell me your story again, and don't leave out any details," or "She finally came out of her depression." At the time, this knowledge helped me see how insidious sense-making was in poetry; even if a poet strained to be dissociative, their brain couldn't help but use coherent image schemas. (In Lautréamont's well-worn conjunction of the surreal, a sewing machine and an umbrella may meet each other, but they do so *on* a dissecting table.) In contemporary poetry that appeared to describe impossible scenes, basic sense lurked in the lines, spatial views appearing like the outlines of old shipwrecks buried under sand. Image schemas functioned as a secret cognitive and linguistic glue, holding us together even when we *tried* to linguistically fall apart.

Motherhood now felt like that to me. I knew, consciously, that my own baby desire was far slighter than that of other women I knew, but I had also unconsciously accepted that giving birth would act as a fulcrum, a kind of tipping point. This was not so much about wanting a baby as expecting a life shaped by one. What would my life look like without that central event around which everything else gained interpretive symmetry? No wonder I was bereft. Without realizing it, I had considered motherhood as a kind of automatic meaning-making machine. Now I was exhausted by the prospect that I would have to craft this meaning on terms that would not be immediately or easily understood by people around me.

One response might have been to accept the calamity, and lean into a reorganization of various forms of structural meaning in my life, but I did not have the presence of mind to do this. Instead, I doubled down, in a panic-stricken, pell-mell kind of way. The doctor recommended that I wait a month or two before testing again, but even if my FSH were to lower and the stimulation protocol were to work, it was unlikely I'd produce a high enough number of eggs to guarantee later pregnancy. (There is a substantial rate of attrition between removal, freezing, re-thawing, fertilization, and implantation: a woman can start out with 25 harvested eggs and end up only with 3 or 4 embryos, and I was most certainly not going to start out with 25.) They suggested that rather than freezing my eggs, I consider freezing embryos, or better still, using fresh embryos then and there. That was the best way to guarantee a pregnancy. Of course, there was the small matter of finding sperm and a person willing to be a father too.

I didn't blink. Rather than step back, I ran forward, further into the world of reproductive technologies, headfirst into an attempt to fall pregnant, not by sex, but by laparoscope and micropipette and catheter tube. If this sounds like a remarkable escalation of events, it was. IVF will do that to you. I was not calm. I was not deliberate. I was not trained for this kind of expedition. Those who are reading this and who have gone through this experience will probably read it quickly, barely blinking. Those who are more removed might well be appalled. *How did she let this happen? How have we gotten to the point where this is considered an appropriate course of action?* There are many answers to those questions, and none of them are comfortable.

PAPER, SPOON, CYST

To see your insides with your own eyes—rather than simply to possess them unconsciously and involuntarily—is a remarkably recent development. Until the beginning of the twentieth century, you could not look inside yourself while you were alive. For centuries, to see even the naked outside of a body, particularly a woman's, was a charged event. There are a number of obvious reasons why. If a ciswoman's body was spectacle (and most of Western art would agree), there was power in restricting its availability. In marriage, it was often the husband who would determine a wife's display. Shame was a mark of control and value.

In Europe, before seeing was listening. Until 1750, doctors tended to rely heavily on the patient's own narrative of their sickness, keeping (to a modern eye) what looks like a remarkable physical distance. They rarely asked the patient to undress. They might touch insofar as they measured the pulse, noted the skin (clammy or hot), and examined the urine and stool, but palpation was thought to have limited use beyond specific tumors. They did not operate, did not cut the skin; that was the work of surgeon-barbers, who were looked down upon for developing knowledge in the hands rather than the mind. Doctors prided themselves on the intellectual agility of their various diagnoses; physical distance was a marker of perceptiveness. Their listening was so labor-intensive that sometimes they only visited two or three patients a day.

Vestigial traces of this kind of intensive listening occur today. In IVF, it's the first chapter of care. In the clinics I attended, the first introductory appointment was always in the doctor's office, with no equipment in it at all. It was a room for listening, the desk between us insistently symbolic. "Tell me," each doctor said, pen poised over paper. I looked at their faces as they listened to me speak. I barely remember the first doctor, but the second doctor's face was mild, wide open, oddly unlined. He didn't look like he'd been angry much, or even disappointed. I decided this was a good thing. It was obvious, by the movement of their pens, that the doctors were both listening for numbers, and so I adjusted my narration accordingly. My age. Period of infertility. How many miscarriages. How many abortions. How many pregnancies. I tried not to cry, and wondered if other patients tried to keep their grief from their doctor's gate.

This appointment was an "out-of-pocket" expense for which I needed to pay hundreds of dollars; the cost seemed to quietly function as proof of economic privilege (in case my health insurance wouldn't kick in later). I did not know then that this was the longest time I would spend with the doctor, that this was the only time he would sit across from me and listen, at such length, to my words.

In 1760, the Austrian physician Leopold Auenbrugger published an account of his seven years working in the Spanish Hospital in Vienna, where most of his patients were soldiers. He had developed a method of tapping on a patient's chest to determine if their lungs were filled with liquid or air, which he later confirmed at autopsy. Thirty years later, in Paris, Jean-Nicolas Corvisart experimented with Auenbrugger's methods and learned to identify certain disorders of the heart by placing his hand against the rib cage and assessing its vibration. One of his students, René Laennec, adopted the practice of applying his ear to the patient's chest to listen to the heart and lungs. When he encountered a patient in 1816 with suspected heart failure, he could not get close enough to the heart because of her breasts. Out of circumspection and frustration, he hit upon the idea of rolling some paper into a tube, and applying that to her chest. The heart's percussive sounds were clearly amplified. This was the first stethoscope: created to circumvent a woman's breasts, her flesh.

The stethoscope possessed few acoustic advantages over the older technique of applying one's ear directly to the patient's chest, but it clarified diagnosis and offered distance—not just from women's bodies, but also from the poor in public hospitals, who filled the wards as they moved from the country to the city in France, swept up in the larger geographic redistributions of the Industrial Revolution. Many suffered from a host of acute infectious and chronic diseases. Their numbers revolutionized methods of clinical diagnosis: in Paris alone, by 1830, there were thirty hospitals containing a total of 20,000 patients. Doctors could see thousands of cases of the same disease—and could accordingly specialize. Clinical notetaking became systematized. Statistics could now be applied to the study of medicine. According to Malcolm Nicolson, the stethoscope "began a process by which the basis of the understanding of disease was taken away from the patient and invested in signs and symbols that were accessible and intelligible only to the doctor. . . . Disease was no longer understood principally in terms of symptoms experienced by the patient but in terms of structural changes detected by an examining physician." The patient was no longer an expert on their own sickness. Doctors learned to listen to the body, not to its words.

The stethoscope and the standardization and systematization of medical care helped construct a hierarchy of perception and shame, a minute set of social distinctions about when it was acceptable to transgress, or what transgression was more acceptable than another. If not verbal speech, then touch—but better touching without sight than touching with it. In Barbara Duden's study of women who consulted the eighteenth-century German physician Johann Storch, she noted that Storch's patients spoke frankly about genital and menstrual matters, but virtually refused to be touched. They agreed to being palpated in the near-dark. In 1839, a doctor in Edinburgh called James Young Simpson developed a uterine sound, a metal probe that could be used to assess the presence of tumors or obstructions. It was made of silver, and about nine inches long with an ivory handle. Young's instructions to other doctors were very explicit: at all costs, the body must be covered when using the uterine sound. Do it, he wrote, with the patient in bed and under a sheet. If you exposed her, it was "at your peril both as a practitioner and gentleman." One husband in Paris in 1839 went so far as to photograph the boil on his wife's midsection, and show the doctor the image rather than allow him to examine her body. A follow-up photograph was taken to evaluate her progress. Instinctively, representation was thought to hold less shame than the flesh itself.

I can imagine you reading this, listening, turning the page, curling the paper, establishing your own distance, relying on my words rather than my body. Here is a representation, not the thing itself: here is what I'm willing to show you. I am minimizing my shame, unsure of my own amplification.

JAMES MARION SIMS, the man who would one day be called the father of modern gynecology, was born in 1813, in Lancaster County, South Carolina. His father—who had been a laborer, surveyor, accountant, and bookkeeper, kept the village hotel, and served as a sheriff before fighting in the Revolutionary War—wanted his son to pick one profession, and stick to it. Sims had three options: law, the church, or medicine. Faced with an indifferent performance as an undergraduate, Sims didn't have the grades for law, and in good conscience knew he wasn't meant for the church. That left medicine— the least desirable of the three. His father didn't mince his words: "It is a profession for which I have the utmost contempt. [. . .] There is no honor to be achieved in it; no reputation to be made, and to think that *my* son should be going around from house to house through the country, with a box of pills in one hand and a squirt in the other, to ameliorate human suffering, is a thought I never supposed I should have to contemplate." The field had barely "professional-ized": the scientific periodical *The Lancet* (and with it, a standard for collective medical opinion) began in 1823, little more than a decade before Sims graduated. By his own account, Sims's year and a half of medical school was nearly useless, and he returned home to South Carolina to set up practice with, in his words, "no clinical advantages." His first patients were two babies that died of diarrhea, and the experience of caring for them was so traumatic that he threw his own business sign down a well, convinced that he could not continue. Medicine, he wrote, was heroic, but it was also murderous; he thought it obvious that it was better to "trust entirely to nature than to . . . doctors." Unlike others, he avoided bleeding his patients, prescribed as little medicine as possible, and kept his hands unusually clean.

More than fifty years later, Sims published the imaginatively titled *The Story of My Life*, which focused on the various surgical techniques and devices that he developed over the course of his career, particularly those that helped women conceive, including artificial insemination and cervical surgery. One such device that Sims claimed to invent was the speculum, though similar devices had been developed in the Roman Empire and referred to in multiple books throughout the sixteenth and seventeenth century. (That Sims didn't know this perhaps reveals how much a standard of knowledge in gynecology had not been established among male medical doctors.)

Anyone who has had a pap smear in this century knows what the speculum is; it now looks like a prosthetic duck bill or an esoteric kitchen implement designed to crush nuts. It is a device used for inspecting the cervix and interior walls of the vagina. It pries the walls of the vaginal cavity open, and holds them apart. And any doctor with a good bedside manner will try to narrate to you what is happening as they use it. *I'm just inserting the speculum now*, they'll say, and you'll feel a penetration of cold metal. *Now I'm opening it up.* The object inside you will widen and bloom, and your body will be pushed apart just a little bit more. You'll hear a clicking noise as they lock it into place. When they release the speculum and remove it, there is a sudden ease, a bodily relief.

Sim's account of how he invented the speculum is told with genuine enthusiasm and excitement. By 1845, he had spent a decade building a substantial medical practice in Montgomery, Alabama. On one visit to a slaveholder's estate, he found a woman in labor for more than seventy-two hours. The baby had died, still within her pelvis, and he removed it with forceps. A week later, he was called back to the estate; the mother was bleeding, and large tears in her perineum allowed urine and feces to circulate freely between her bladder, anus, and vagina. She had what was and is now called a vesicovaginal fistula. It meant she was both incontinent and prone to suffering from infection—and that meant, to her slaveholder, that she was losing her value.

Sims identified this vesicovaginal fistula at the same time that slaveholders began to understand the value in producing more enslaved children. Before 1807, and the Act Prohibiting Importation of Slaves, it was cheaper for slaveholders to buy new enslaved people than it was to allow the ones they already had to give birth. Slaveholders felt it was entirely within their rights to disrupt any nascent relationships between the enslaved by selling one person on. Many women also resisted bringing new life into servitude. But by the 1830s, it was well established that the best way for slaveholders to increase their holdings was to multiply rather than buy. By 1860, the African-American population in the United States had increased to almost 4 million—a 3.5 million increase in less than a century, and due almost entirely to a birth rate of 9 to 10 children per woman, despite an infant mortality of more than twice the rate of white mothers, and despite the fact that abortion and miscarriage were reported widely among populations of enslaved women. Although the United States only accounted for 6 percent of the enslaved people imported from Africa worldwide, by 1860 it accounted for more than 60 percent of the Northern Hemisphere's enslaved population.

In other words, what appears to be a curious rash of incidents of vesicovaginal fistula in Sims's book—shortly after examining one enslaved woman, another slaveholder contacted him with a similar case, and then another—was also the result of a population explosion that Sims does not name. He only incidentally informs us in his book that he built a "slave hospital" in his backyard which had eight beds, and that he owned enslaved medical attendants.

In *The Story of My Life*, Sims notes that around the same time he saw these first cases of vesicovaginal fistula, he also saw another patient, a white woman of means, who had fallen from her horse and had somehow "retroverted" her uterus. Sims describes at length the position he put her in (resting on her knees) so he could touch her uterus. He realized if he put one of the women suffering from a tear in her vagina in the same position, and inserted a spoon of some kind to press apart the walls of the vagina, he might be able to see their wound more clearly. If you can see a problem, apparently, you can fix it. He rushed to the hardware store, purchasing a set of spoons, and returned to his hospital where he asked a woman called Betsey, his second case of vesicovaginal fistula, to kneel on a table and put her head on the palm of her hands. Two medical students held her down, and pulled the cheeks of her buttocks apart. "Introducing the bent handle of the spoon I saw everything, as no man had ever seen before," he wrote later. "The walls of the vagina could be seen closing in every direction; the neck of the uterus was distinct and well-defined, and even the secretions from the neck could be seen as a tear glistening in the eye, clear even and distinct, as plain as could be." Sims the gynecological explorer: it was as if he had entered a new valley system, and was charting the terrain. Betsey's fistula was now obvious, as was the fact that it was "simply" a tear that could be mended with stitches, like any other wound. Filled with enthusiasm, Sims notified slaveholders in the surrounding area that he would house and feed any enslaved woman suffering from a fistula so that he could develop and refine a surgical procedure to fix it. Six or seven more women arrived. He built a second floor on his slave hospital. He expected to cure them in six months.

It took five years. Sims found that he could close up sections of a tear, but smaller holes remained, and the seepage continued regardless of their size. His use of silk thread, then wire, caused extensive infections, as did his use of sponges left inside these women post-surgery, which were supposed to absorb urine. He did not use anesthesia, though he did give women opium for weeks after each operation. Some of these women endured up to thirty operations. After a couple of years, the Montgomery doctors stopped attending. Their reservations, Sims reported, had to do with the economic burden of housing the patients, as well as the strain his work schedule placed on his family—all told, he had nine children with his wife, Theresa Sims (née Jones). If there were any ethical concerns, Sims didn't mention them. His patients became his assistants, the women holding each other down. The briefness of his descriptions of their pain is heartbreaking. "Lucy's agony was extreme," he writes. "She was much prostrated, and I thought she was going to die." But she didn't. She went on to endure multiple operations. Sims does not mention, though his protégé, Nathan Bozeman, later noted that the surgery only cured half of the African American women in his practice. When Sims decided to move from Montgomery to Butler

Springs for his health, he took three enslaved women on whom to continue practicing.

Eventually, he moved to New York City, where his clientele, but not his rationale, changed. In Montgomery, he had been able to carve out a practice by tending to African Americans, both free and enslaved, and later, the city's Jewish population. When he moved to New York City, which was crowded with medical practitioners, he took on the working-class end of the market, and founded a hospital for poor women. You could call this generosity—and I'm sure to some degree it was. But it was also a pragmatic positioning, which he acknowledged. He had to make a professional impression, and he did so by also becoming known for a variety of surgical devices and techniques that would cure infertility. Many of his theories were not sound, to say the least. He thought you could increase the chances of conception by making cuts in the cervix with a scalpel, which would allow sperm to move through. For women who suffered from "vaginismus," which was an instinctive contraction of the vagina that made sex impossible, he administered anesthetic, allowing their husbands to have sex with them. But other parts of his account remain uneasily resonant. He was particularly proud of an examination chair he had built, and printed the specifications in his autobiography along with diagrams. With it, he noted, a (white) woman could sit upright and be gently reclined, easing the social transition (and what it implied) between the vertical and the horizontal.

I have sat on those chairs. Anyone who has undergone a pap smear or cervical exam has. Sims's treatment of middle-class white infertility only came after he had specialized in enslaved Black fertility. The "dignity" of a white female patient has been at the cost of a Black woman's suffering.

In his autobiography, Sims did not reflect on the difference between his respect for his white patients' dignity and his positioning of Betsey and other enslaved women. He does not reflect on his choice to withhold anesthetic from his African American patients, but administer it to his white ones. He does not think about the fact that "the dread of my young life," as he writes "was mad dogs and 'runaway n_____'" [my redaction]. It's a throwaway line. He does not explain because he feels no need. Even if he fantasizes about what harm an African American might do to him, he does not think about how this fear may have deadened his empathy for another human being. It's not that Sims lacked self-reflection, or did not care about how he appeared to others. In his book, he took great pains to establish that his move to New York was because of his health, rather than any particular ambition. To him, the publication of articles about surgical procedures was simply the scholarly sharing of knowledge: his establishment of the women's hospital was the only way to break into the market. Over and over again he wrote that he had to be talked into these schemes by supporters. His modesty is so persistent that it is a textual tic. He is terrified of hubris. It is revealing, therefore, that Sims was never defensive about his treatment of African American women.

In this context, Sims was not remarkable at all. In the nineteenth century, doctors throughout the United States conducted experiments on enslaved people that they would not have dreamed of inflicting on their white patients; half of the original articles in the 1836 *Southern Medical and Surgical Journal* dealt with experiments performed on African Americans. Some of these nineteenth-century experiments are well documented; 30 of the first 37 experimental cesarean surgeries performed by François Marie Prevost were on

African American patients. Others were more-private exercises in sadism. In the freedom seeker John Brown's memoir, *Slave Life in Georgia*, Brown recalls being forced to sit naked in a pit of hot embers until he passed out, so that a Dr. Thomas Hamilton of Clinton, Georgia, could assess the effects of heat stroke. Dr. Hamilton also flayed Brown to see how "deep" his darkness went. Then there were the experiments, Brown wrote, "which I cannot dwell upon."

Sims's medical ethics may seem clearly removed from our own sense of reproductive potential or history, but unethical medical experimentation on African American people continued long past Sims's era; he is only remarkable in that he narrated it with such vigor. As Harriet Washington makes clear in her book *Medical Apartheid*, late into the twentieth century the medical industry in the United States regularly used disproportionately large numbers of African Americans in medical trials, particularly in those that posed a substantial risk to the patient. This is not just the 1932–1972 Tuskegee Syphilis Study, in which over four hundred African American men weren't informed they had contracted syphilis, and were merely observed for twenty-five years without being treated. Washington has persuasively documented a systemic indifference to African American pain that continues today, even if there has been a tidal shift regarding the more generalized sense of moral outrage we know we ought to feel. It was only in 2018 that the statue of Sims, which stood on the border of Central Park, across the road from the New York Academy of Medicine, was removed. A more liberalized political agenda, even if it is just political correctness, has sensitized us to the cruder forms of racist rhetoric. But it has also encouraged us to compartmentalize the problem: Sims's problem was supposedly with African American women, and not related to his abilities as a surgeon or his view of female patients and their "capacities." His insensitivity is attributed to his racism, rather than his misogyny or medical training, yet each quality appears to have enabled the others.

AT THE END of my first IVF consultation with my doctor, he told me he would need to look at my uterus and follicles and led me to another room. He told me to undress completely, to make sure the opening of the paper gown was at the front, then left me alone for five minutes. This was done before they had drawn any blood, and before they knew my FSH results.

I immediately recognized the ultrasound machine next to the chair. In movies and television shows, it has become a synecdoche for people confronting the reality of a pregnancy: one moving image inside another moving image, film reflexively claiming its own generative power. The actors hush, examine the screen with awe. The wand circles over the stomach, slipping on the gel, then halts, presses gently: There! A life! The heartbeat flickers rapidly, keeping its own time against the swaying, pulsing uterus. It's become so ubiquitous that people now announce a pregnancy with an ultrasound still, so ubiquitous that I tried not to look directly at the machine. The grief that flowed from my uncertainty about what was to come was a river thick and wide.

When the doctor returned five minutes later, it was with a phalanx of others, nurses or physicians' assistants, who busied themselves around the room, turning on screens, pulling out clipboards, dimming the lights even further. I was asked to put my legs in stirrups. The doctor told me to move my hips further down the table.

I wiggled a little, the paper rustling beneath me. "No, a few more inches," he said. "A few more." He waited. "Closer. No. Closer." I kept on insufficiently wiggling, and he kept on patiently repeating himself.

I thought of Norbert Elias, the sociologist who suggested that one marker of civilization is a shift from external sanctions to internal self-control. According to his reasoning, the more shame you felt, the more civilized you were. Was my shame a marker of civilization? If so, I was impressed by how quickly I was rearranging my conceptual categories of revelation: I was reclassifying, on the hoof, a medical exam that would otherwise be considered an indignity. The chair, its slow recline, my wriggle, was a way to perform passivity and consent. This was conceived by Sims as a *gift* to his female patients, a form of respect: if we know the transition will be difficult, one option is to draw it out, frame it, so that we all have time to understand and identify the boundary enough to push past it. In past centuries, a shared conception of shame could paradoxically create the necessary conditions under which a ciswoman *would* permit a physician to examine her: it could be generally agreed that it must have been necessary, rather than desirable. The same went for me now. These doctors and nurses who saw me now probably knew I was embarrassed. They may have been a little embarrassed, but they'd done it so many times it only registered in the formality of their tone.

I had been told that I was to have a transvaginal ultrasound, but I didn't quite realize what that was until I watched a doctor cover a long slender white dildoesque probe with a plastic sheath. All the while narrating his actions, he inserted it into my vagina, and pushed it inside. "This should only be a slight pressure," he said, eyes flickering to my face, then on to the screen next to him. The symbolism of this kind of ultrasound felt humiliating. How was this *not* supposed to be a penetration? How was I supposed to *not* react to this? By contrast, a pregnancy ultrasound now felt like a benediction. I tried to still my face. Everyone was looking there, at my body, on the screen, which was tilted so that I could see it too.

"This is your uterus," he said. "I'm going to measure your uterine lining, to see how thick it is." He started to call out numbers, clicking crosshairs over sections of the image. One of the nurses wrote the numbers down on the clipboard.

"Is it thick enough?" I asked.

"Looks good to me. Now we're going to look at your ovaries, and see how many follicles are in each." He pushed the wand to the left, and circles of light swam into view. The follicles were black dots, droplets of balsamic vinegar. I was fascinated by how dark they were, how distinct. My body was juddering, twitching with life. If you can see a problem, you can fix it. I don't remember how many he counted that first time.

Ultrasound technology was first developed in the 1950s by a British surgeon called Ian Donald. At that time, surgery was the only way to determine the nature of a lump, and that had obvious risks. Donald had a background in radio and sonar from his service during the war, and understood the basics of ultrasound, which had been developed in World War II as a way to detect microscopic flaws in boat hulls using sonar. He suspected that ultrasound might be able to distinguish between different types of soft tissue, which an X-ray could not do. Even more promisingly, Donald knew that while sonar technology could cause side effects similar to those of radiography and nuclear medicine, ultrasound could diminish this cellular perturbation to a fraction of what a patient experienced during an X-ray.

When Donald took up a research position at the University of Glasgow, he began a series of experiments at a local engineering firm's research department; he was interested to see if their industrial detecting equipment (used to locate flaws in metal welds) could distinguish between different types of tissue. In an article written for the *Annals of the Royal College of Surgeons of England* twenty years later, he recalled taking one summer's afternoon to find out if the machine could differentiate between beefsteak, human fibroid, and cyst. He had tucked each kind of tissue inside the other, but there on the screen were distinct markers of sound: "A cyst produced echoes only at depth from the near and far walls, whereas a solid tumour progressively attenuated echoes at increasing depths of penetration." With Tom Brown, a research engineer, he set about building a series of diagnostic prototypes that could be tried out on patients in Glasgow Hospital.

Donald was a man with a sense of humor. He later recounted the problems of his earliest prototypes; one of the first devices could only see material at least 8 cm away, so they had to develop a system of buckets filled with water to naturally extend the probe's distance. It was not easy to position all this equipment, and many patients ended up lying in very wet beds. To avoid more spills, they tried putting the water in balloons, and settled on condoms as the ideal sheath. A friend from out of town agreed to buy the condoms and save Donald the infamy (a consideration in 1950s Glasgow). Donald recalled that "asked whether he wanted plain or teat ended condoms he [the friend] said he did not know but would run out to the car and find out." This story soon received city-wide circulation.

Over the next few years, as they developed new prototypes in conjunction with engineers, Donald and his colleagues became adept at interpreting vague and blurred images. But it did not occur to him to use ultrasound to determine fetal health. Rather, a staff nurse called Marjorie Marr in the maternity ward started to borrow the machine to determine the positioning of the baby if the patient was judged obese. Donald realized that if the position of the head could be readily determined, it must be quite possible to evaluate the fetus's growth, and one could begin to systematize expected milestones of growth and development. Donald followed Marr's lead. By 1963, he was using ultrasound to evaluate the uterus (rather than just the fetal head), and a year later, diagnosing early pregnancies of 6 to 7 weeks, identifying the egg sac and the fetal pole. Once he had presented his results to multiple obstetric societies and hospitals, it was only a matter of time before other companies began to develop ultrasound probes for commercial use in medicine. By the 1970s, ultrasound departments were being established in hospitals throughout the United Kingdom and beyond.

It is remarkable how quickly ultrasound machines became ubiquitous in fetal medicine and new reproductive technologies; no one thinks twice now about the verification of life as image. It might be because, on some level, things haven't really changed: an ultrasound is precisely that; a set of sound waves that discerns differentiations in tissue, which is then translated into an image. What we were all looking at in that examination room was a sound. We are still living in the age of the stethoscope, not so far away from James Young Simpson and his uterine probe as we like to think. Tom Brown, the engineer who developed medical ultrasound, wasn't permitted to operate his machine on patients for fear of impropriety; he had to watch, at a distance, as a medically qualified "operator" produced the images. (It was so difficult to determine whether an unclear image was due to the machine or to its operator that Brown set about developing an automatic scanner, which could adjust and anticipate according to the contours of the body.) I don't think it's any accident that the examining rhythm of the IVF visit—narration, dimmed lights, sound as sight—mimics the consultative emphases of the past three hundred years. We are heard, then translated: into numbers we cannot understand, watching sounds as images. In our eagerness to look inside, we forget how much modern medicine descends from a tradition of keeping the body at a clothed distance. We have learned how to hold the body far from us, still expecting to look inside, to discover the vast intimacy of a world within a world. This looking inside is so often looking away.

When my doctor was done, he removed the plastic sheath from the wand out of my line of sight, along with his gloves. I heard the bin lid clang. I was told to take my time dressing, and then they all left me to gather myself together.

TWO YEARS AFTER that first transvaginal ultrasound, I sat in my doctor's office, across the small table from him. I had never returned to this room during my treatment, but now I was there to talk about this book. He had agreed to give me an hour of his time, no charge. "Tell me," I wanted to say, and I wanted to listen. I can hear his voice right now, writing this. It's like his face: easy, quiet, methodical.

He had entered reproductive medicine in the 1980s, when it was a new field with a huge amount of potential; the rate of fertilization could be (and was) improved. It was a specialty in which you could make a difference. He spoke of intersections: medicine and the humanities, obstetrics and endocrinology, surgery and medicine. He wasn't so much driven by the subject of infertility as much as by the fact that the field was a good structural fit for him. It had both clinical and research dimensions. Working in a field that was growing so much was one way to keep the emotional weight of the work at bay. He gave me a list of organizations, journals, and conference proceedings to review, a list of key people in the field. He had been practicing for more than three decades, immersed in a field I had only just stumbled into.

As he spoke, it became clear: Auenbrugger would be beside the point to him. So would Corvisart and Laennec. So would Sims. Or rather—so far beyond the point that led him to sit on the other side of that small table. There are three distinct strains of literature on reproductive medicine: medical literature, accounts by people who've experienced it (and their communication with each other), and feminist anthropology and medical history. They do not connect as much as you might expect: their respective audiences do not tend to coincide. I found myself not wanting to ask him what he thought about the thousands upon thousands of women posting on internet message boards about their experiences of infertility. I did not ask him about FINRRAGE, the Feminist International Network of Resistance to Reproductive and Genetic Engineering which was formed in 1985, which argued that countries needed to reject reproductive technologies, or at least stringently review them. I did not ask him about the marked gender imbalance in reproductive technologies in particular: most doctors are cismale; nearly all nurses are cisfemale. I did not ask him why he thought IVF nursing has the second-highest turnover rate of any specialty (topped only by oncology). I did not ask him if it worried him that IVF and technologies like it only seemed to reaffirm the reproductive abilities of the rich and/or the well-insured in the United States, or that the distinct majority of his patients were white, or that the basic premise of most of the protocols he administered for male-factored infertility involved surgical interventions for women. I did not ask him about anthropological or sociological or cultural studies understandings of IVF. I did not ask him about all the men I had read about in history or all the women, still writing today, who critiqued them, or the paucity of accounts by nonbinary or transgender patients or doctors. I did not ask him about techno-socialist writing in Britain, the ways in which writers had reimagined embryology and reproduction in novels and short stories.

I did not ask him because I thought he might dismiss these questions as oversimplifications, or red herrings, or simply beside the point when one remembered the pain and grief of women who wanted a baby and could not have one. I did not ask him because I understood, anticipated, even supported his dismissals. He was the expert and I was one of those women he had helped. I did not want to bite the hand that gave me a baby. So I went away and continued to gnaw at mine in private.

4

. . .

ALL MY POSTERITY

I t is worth asking why there are extraordinarily few narrative accounts, even by women who have the privilege and freedom to
publish, of their reproductive frame of mind throughout history.

Most of the stories we have are numbers driven, and any sense of
individual motivation is cast like a shadow. In New England in the
sixteenth and seventeenth centuries, the Anglo-American woman
gave birth to eight children on average. If one were to accept that a
woman's fertility declines for about nine months after birth while
she breastfeeds, and factor in a few miscarriages, eight live births
amount to about two decades of constant breastfeeding and/or
gestation. With an average life expectancy of less than forty years at
the time, mothering at this scale was a life's work. Elliptical sentences and brief reports hint at the population explosion. One set-
tler, Elizabeth Appleton, wrote, for example, "of all my posterity. 6
sons and 3 daughters, 20 grand son and 20 grand daughters, 58 in
all. 33 are gon before me. I hope I shall mett them all att Christ's rit
hand among his sheep and lambs" [sic]. Nearly one in four infants
died before their first year, and nearly half of all children did not

survive past their tenth year. One in five women died in childbirth. The general arithmetic seems clear: give birth to double the number of children you want, and pray to God that you survived your first, which was when you found out just how wide your hips were. The risks—of death, grief, illness—were remarkable. By 1751, the European American population was doubling every twenty years, at a rate that the economist Thomas Malthus claimed was "probably without parallel in history." This growth was religious and political: to go forth, be fruitful and multiply was God's bidding, but also necessary if colonies were to continue, let alone thrive.

Those whose actions did not appear to support this reproductive reasoning were considered with suspicion. You were twice as likely to be accused of witchcraft if you had not given birth. If a baby was born stillborn or deformed, or there was a miscarriage, foul spirits and wicked women were suspected. Most of the women accused of witchcraft were also older than forty, which suggests, ironically, that as women reached the biological limits of their fertility, other people suspected they thought about children even more: witches were believed, as the historian John Demos has noted, "to have an inordinate, and envious, interest in infants and small children." (This is also the case in many fairy tales, where a woman's interest in another's children is often explicitly predatory: the witch in "Hansel and Gretel" lives alone and eats up children, and Dame Gothel in "Rapunzel" insists that her neighbors give their daughter to her.) Barrenness was not grounds for divorce, but the refusal to procreate was. In other words, the inability to procreate was less morally subversive than a preference not to.

Explosion, implosion: at the same time that an Anglo-American woman's purpose was defined by her ability to prodigiously reproduce, Native American communities were facing the possibility of complete extinction through genocide, starvation, and diseases for which they had no immunity. Their reproductive rates collapsed. Before the arrival of Columbus in 1492, there were probably around 7 million Native Americans living in the United States area. (Estimates range between 2.1 and 18 million.) By the nineteenth century, that number had been reduced by more than 90 percent, to 600,000.

Time and again in American history, some groups have been exhorted to reproduce, and others actively discouraged, if not denied. In President Theodore Roosevelt's sixth annual message to Congress in 1903, he warned that "There are regions in our own land, and classes of our population, where the birth rate has sunk below the death rate. . . . No man, no woman, can shirk the primary duties of life, whether for love of ease and pleasure, or for any other cause, and retain his or her self-respect." Roosevelt's comments were part of an increasingly vocal eugenics movement in the United States, which had political, clerical, medical, and cultural proponents in the highest positions of authority. They were worried, as one physician put in the *Ladies Home Journal*, about "race suicide among the rich." They blamed immigrants from southern, central, and eastern Europe for the weakening of the social fabric and picked out vice zones and amusement centers, moral experimentation, and class and racial mixing as obvious harbingers of societal destruction. The obstetrician George B. H. Swayze wrote: "The *patriotic* [my emphasis] enterprise of recruiting [the] American population with the blood of American citizenship is being gradually shifted to the lusty sexual output of foreign breeders. . . . The Jew, the Russian, the Hungarian, the Italian complexion is to-day darkly outshading the

Americanized descendants of the English, the Irish, and Scotch, the German and Swede" [sic]. Swayze's racial othering was a kind of reproductive whack-a-mole in the service of perpetuating an Anglo-Saxon Protestant Whiteness. He continued: "This backward lapse of national progress hinges on the fact that our educated, restless, esthetic American women have preached to womanhood the subtleties of emulating manhood in the guise of worldly spheres, and have developed among the masses an ethical, almost a constitutional reluctance to pregnancy." The highest rate of childlessness in women was among the college-educated, which led a physician to write in 1919: "Prevent young girls from over-studying." Roosevelt admonished (white) women to think of their reproductive abilities in the same way that men thought about military service: as a form of patriotism, a higher calling. In 1914, Congress established Mother's Day as a public holiday to express "our love and reverence for the mothers of our country," one of many efforts to legally sanctify the role of motherhood.

I grew up almost eight thousand miles away from the United States (in Aotearoa, we would call it twelve and a half thousand kilometers), but my ancestors were English, Irish, and Scottish settlers, soldiers, doctors, bridge builders, photographers, and shipmakers, who had large families of nine, even eleven children, in a land where Māori were also facing the possibility of extinction through war, forced resettlement, and the introduction of diseases for which they had no immunity. Māori reproductive rates collapsed at precisely the time that my colonial ancestors' began to thrive. Pre-contact, in the eighteenth century, there were probably between 100,000 and 200,000 Māori living in Aotearoa. In an 1858 census, there were about 60,000.

My childhood and teenage years were spent in a middle-class suburb in the largest city in New Zealand. I am the daughter of an atheist biologist and an Anglican family physician. Though I attended an Anglican school until the age of twelve, I could have counted on the fingers of one hand the people I knew who regularly attended church of any kind. Any sense of white religious racial manifest destiny had been carefully buried under a fierce commitment to egalitarianism and mateship, and feminism was never a dirty word, nor even a particularly loaded one. In New Zealand, we thought of American culture as an overwrought, embarrassing, riveting spectacle—and our own, by comparison, as an exercise in understated humor and plain reason. We did not burn witches. We insisted on a distinction between deliberate genocide and genocidal practices. We celebrated Mother's Day, and didn't think twice about where the custom came from, or when it began.

When we think of our own personal reproductive histories, we tend to detach our own choices from the patterns of centuries of others with the practiced ease of someone tearing off a paper towel: that was then, but this is *me*. Those numbers seem so high, the punishments so extreme. The pressures are so starkly rendered they do not feel real.

So LET ME TRY ANOTHER WAY, and sketch out the negative space: the children that could've been. We've come to think of the exponential increase in women using oral contraceptives in the early 1960s and the legalization of abortion in the United States in 1973 as the beginning of a new era of reproductive choice, but people have always tried to control and direct their reproductive capacity. In

1800, the average married couple in the United States had 7 children, but by 1850, the number had dropped to 5 or 6, and by 1900, to 3 or 4. In less than a century, family sizes *halved*.

J. Marion Sims's career coincided with this time period, but in *The Story of My Life*, he is strikingly silent about family planning, both abortion and birth control. When he started out as a doctor, abortion was legal, and growing increasingly popular. It's been estimated that at the beginning of the nineteenth century, there was 1 abortion for every 25 to 35 live births, and by the middle of the century, the ratio had increased to 1 abortion for every 6 live births. The most dramatic birth rate drop was among the middle class, who were changing their minds about what children were for. For those who had settled in cities and towns, there was no longer the need to have multiple hands to help in the field. The professionalization of multiple vocations meant that it took longer to train. The length of childhood increased. If a child was to get a fair go at life, there needed to be an emphasis on the quality of each child's upbringing, rather than the quantity you were able to produce. In 1878, the Michigan Board of Health estimated that in their state, *one in three pregnancies* ended in abortion, and that most were obtained by "prosperous and otherwise respectable married women." As a young doctor who increasingly specialized in gynecological issues, Sims must have been carrying out abortions for half his career; given his financial worries, which he emphasizes repeatedly, it seems unlikely he would have turned down such lucrative trade. He is also quiet about contraception. The diaphragm was patented in the 1840s, and pessaries, sponges, condoms, and syringes for douching were all available for purchase. By the late nineteenth century, Charles Knowlton's 1832 book on the various forms of birth control was still selling more than 250,000 copies a year. Tellingly, Sims does not discuss it even to denounce it; by 1888, when he published his auto-biography, under the Comstock Act of 1873 it was illegal to send birth control devices or information through the mail. From 1860 to 1890, forty states enacted anti-abortion laws, and by 1900, as May notes, "abortion was a criminal offense in virtually every jurisdiction" in the United States. If Sims's career happened to chart the rise of modern gynecology, it also silently encompassed the rise and fall of abortion and contraception as legal forms of family planning.

Sims's silence was the norm, and if someone broke it, they were punished. In 1911, a woman wrote a letter to *Good Housekeeping* magazine stating she had been married seven years and had deliberately avoided having children. She was extremely happy with her decision, she wrote, and described her friends with children as haggard, worn out, or dead. The response was swift and overwhelmingly negative; of the hundreds of letters written in reply over the next year, only *one* was supportive. The rest thought her letter an apostasy. The cognitive dissonance is remarkable: as family sizes decreased, natalism only grew stronger, more virulent. The writers of those letters to *Good Housekeeping* had all chosen to have fewer children than their mothers, who had, in turn, had fewer children than their grandmothers. Childlessness steadily increased for the first four decades of the twentieth century—certainly affected by the First World War and the Great Depression, but consistently moving downward rather than spiking in reaction to each economic and military calamity. Privately, women and men knew there was a cost to childbearing and acted accordingly, even if they might castigate those who refused to reproduce. By the mid-1920s, the birth rate had dropped to around 2 children per woman.

There were voices of protest. In 1907, "Anonymous, New York City" was heartbreakingly explicit as she pointed out in a letter to the progressive weekly magazine *The Independent* the hypocrisy of the state in encouraging women to have children, but refusing to offer competent medical care, paid maternity leave, or daycare options. She wrote that she had always wanted to be a mother, and her husband wanted a child too. "We have discussed its possibilities, its education, its future," she wrote. "But we have never dared to have it." As Elaine Tyler May has pointed out, "This woman's concern was not with the low birthrate of the educated elite, but the reproductive habits of the American-born working class." The letter writer noted that 12 percent of the population owned 71 percent of the wealth. Why should she bring a child into the world that was "destined," she wrote, "from birth for wage slavery and exploitation?" She concluded her letter addressing the pronatalist elite: "Now gentlemen, You Who Rule Us, we are your 'wage slaves,' my husband and I. . . . You can refuse us any certainty of work, wages or provision for old age. We cannot help ourselves. But there is one thing you cannot do. You cannot use me to breed food for your factories."

It was a remarkable denunciation, and the letter writer's determination is thrown into strong relief when you read *Motherhood in Bondage*, the birth control activist Margaret Sanger's collection of first-person narratives by American women unable to obtain birth control. Hundreds of women had written to Sanger throughout the 1920s seeking counsel, isolated and denied help by their friends, husbands, priests, physicians, and neighbors. The book derives its effect from a monotony of pain: the letter writer usually records the age at which she was married (fifteen, sixteen, nineteen), lists the children she had, then documents the ill effects of not being able to practice reproductive choice: her ill health, botched illegal abortions, the remorseless descent into poverty, children born horrifically underweight, those that couldn't sit up at nineteen months old, husbands who refused to practice abstinence or withdrawal. Though Sanger arranged the letters into chapters of different themes ("Girl Mothers," "The Pinch of Poverty," "The Trap of Maternity," etc.), many of the letters could be swapped from one chapter to another to no ill effect. This letter is entirely typical: "I am forty years old, had eleven children. The oldest twenty-three is feeble-minded, seven died when small, but the oldest takes more care than the three others together. Two years ago I had dropsy when the last baby was born and the doctor told me I had to look out so I would not have any more as it would kill me, but the doctor was not allowed to tell me how to keep out of it, so you see I live in constant fear, so please have pity on me and tell me what to do as I have to live for the children's sake" [sic]. Sanger's argument was crystal clear: contraception offered an increased quality of life to both a mother and her children. It was the humane thing to do.

Growing up in New Zealand, in a metropolitan bubble of middle-class kids, birth control was so readily available that some of my friends were prescribed it for their acne. None of us came from large families. I can't remember a single instance of my parents, relatives, or friends telling me what it would be like when I got married or had a baby. I grew up spending afternoons in the waiting room of my mother's medical practice, or at my father's office at the University of Auckland's medical school, confident of what my flesh was, of where I came from, a collection of cells rather than a soul. The value of science was familial. My aunt, a graphic designer, drew cartoons and anatomical illustrations for a book, *It's OK to Be You!*, about reproductive health for teenagers, which, as a nine-year-old, I took to school to show my friends. (It was deemed slightly *too* mature, and my parents were called.) The knowledge that the women writing to Sanger so desperately needed was easily available to me: my own blood taught it, treated it, illustrated it. I developed, as Swayze put it, a "constitutional reluctance" toward pregnancy. The pressure to do that kind of thing felt deeply external: I tended to dismiss it as a convention I didn't have to follow—like buying a new car, or waxing.

Which is why, perhaps, I never knew how hard it was to actually obtain an abortion in New Zealand, even as I went, effortlessly, onto the pill. English law, applied in 1840, outlawed abortion, and in 1867, New Zealand legislation criminalized anyone who caused a miscarriage. It wasn't until 1974 that the first abortion clinic opened in New Zealand (using vacuum aspiration), and it was raided by police, set on fire by anti-abortion activists, and forced to close for a few years before reopening in 1980. During that time, organizations were set up to fund the costs for women to travel to Australia, where abortions were more easily obtained. Though legislation was passed in 1978 that set out a legal framework for abortion, the hurdles were considerable: women were not allowed to self-refer, and had to see their family doctor and two medical consultants beforehand who would assess the mental and physical grounds for carrying out an abortion.

My mother, working as a family doctor throughout the 1980s and 1990s, spoke to thousands of women seeking a referral. We never spoke about it. On the weekends, she'd occasionally speak on the phone to a patient with an emergency, and I'd hear the way her voice deepened, slowed, grew more precise. Her face took on a watchful look, a little fox-like. She was on the founding committee of the nonprofit Doctors for Sexual Abuse Care (DSAC), which essentially meant she worked on-call to provide immediate medical assessments in cases of sexual assault. She would return home from those shifts, willing to tell me about the people she had seen and evaluated, the evidence she had preserved. I grew up with a fairly graphic understanding of the relationship between sex and trauma, and the legal barriers to me exercising full reproductive choice were quietly tucked away behind other freedoms: they existed, but I never happened to hit them. In New Zealand, it wasn't until 2003 that women were allowed to take mifepristone (an early-pregnancy abortion pill) at home. It wasn't until 2019 that a woman was allowed to privately pursue an abortion without first talking to her family doctor.

I SPENT MY TWENTIES in graduate school, then teaching and writing. I focused, as many women do, on moving outward, beyond the domestic. New York City offered a delayed independence, and it was filled with people who had made similar decisions. We had time to try things out—relationships, neighborhoods, careers. When people I knew had a child, they kept on disappearing, moving upstate or to cheaper cities. This was a release valve that also delayed confrontation. All the while, in both New Zealand and in the United States, history stood far closer to me than I thought it did, its breath on my neck.

I just didn't recognize it as history. Instead, I started to worry. The anxieties were low-grade, but multitudinous. I worried that I had made a mistake, but I worried that I didn't fantasize about smelling babies, or dressing them, or taking them on holiday, or having parent friends. I worried that I didn't want to dote, and I assumed that because I didn't want these things, my desire for a child wasn't genuine. I didn't have a particularly strong maternal instinct. I knew the world was slowly collapsing socially and environmentally, and I felt bad about bringing a child into it, about putting the Earth's needs behind my own. I had a career. I didn't want to sign years of my life over to the needs of another human being, but I also didn't know if I had it in me to create a life that would warrant not having children. My father told me that people had children when they realized their careers weren't going to work out the way they wanted, or that it would take more time and hard work than they wanted to give. I wondered if that was true for me (and for him). I didn't know how I was going to have the time to raise a child. I felt guilty for both wanting children and fearing what they would bring. I worried that wanting kids was a failure of the imagination, a knee-jerk desire, the result of subliminal conditioning, too many rom-coms and matter-of-fact friends. I was worried my desire was suspect because it seemed to rise unbidden, and because I believed that gender was constructed, and how could I unravel what appeared natural when I knew it wasn't? Where would I start? I worried that I wanted kids because I was lonely.

And still, I wanted them. Some people would call this a biological or hormonal urge, or evolutionarily natural. I was and remain unconvinced we should rationalize it this way. As Anna Rotkirch has pointed out, "most parents in human history have had their children before they had the time or opportunity to long for them." When baby longing appears, it tends to be tied to the culturally expected age of birth, rather than any biological demarcation of fertility. It comes when a person senses that in a parallel life, they could have been a parent by now: the opportunity has presented itself, and they have not pursued it. They are grieving a decision they did not make. The age at which this longing appears is culturally subjective and gendered. In different countries, women marry and give birth at different ages: in Tanzania, the average age for first births is nineteen, in India, sixteen. In the United States, it is twenty-seven—precisely the age I moved here. I worried about this concurrence. The anxiety only grew. What felt like doubt was an undercurrent of history still so powerful that it ended up knocking me off my feet.

AT THE END of the Second World War, the declining birth rate began to reverse itself. Between 1946 and 1964, the West experienced a baby boom that was remarkably consistent across all ethnicities and social, occupational, and economic classes. For these two decades, the total number of births exceeded 2 per woman. Probably 12 percent of the population in the United States suffered from infertility at the time, but in surveys, *zero* percent of women said that childlessness was a preferred state. Natalism had reached its apogee. In New Zealand, my grandparents lived through this peak. Both of my parents were born in 1949.

There was, of course, the basic collective joy of having survived the worldwide catastrophe of World War II. Servicemen and women returned home to their countries determined to put the war behind them: to create life, rather than end it, to devote oneself to the structure of a family rather than a military hierarchy. That is, at least, how my paternal grandfather saw it. Grey returned home from fighting in North Africa and Europe, married Val, the younger sister of his best friend, and threw himself into raising four children, even avoiding visits to the local Royal New Zealand Returned and Services' Association, where he could socialize with other veterans. He worked first as a manager of the produce section in a supermarket, and later owned his own produce store. The only stories my grandfather would tell about his time overseas were funny. The one material reminder was a carved wooden cherub's head, taken from the bombed ruins of the Abbey of Monte Cassino in Italy. It sat on the mantelpiece: a child looking back over a ghostly shoulder at my father and his siblings growing up.

Just like her mother before her, my paternal grandmother, Val, worked as a secretary before marriage. Both left their jobs to concentrate on starting a family. I do not know whether they wanted to or not. Bessie, my great-grandmother, had two children, and Val, her daughter, had four. Contraction, expansion, right on cue. I do not know if these were the numbers they wanted. I loved Val fiercely, and we wrote letters to each other every month for more than a decade after I left New Zealand and before she died, but she never spoke of choices she did or didn't make.

With my maternal grandmother, Ro, things were different. She was unhappy enough in life for a few adults to feel they had to explain this fact to me when I was a child. Most attributed it to stymied ambition. She had served as an ambulance driver in the First World War, and was also expected to put that down in order to pick up a family. She had three daughters, and one foundational memory of theirs was her decision to leave them (all younger than six years old) with a nanny when my grandfather received a fellowship to practice medicine in London for a year. As a child, I remember her sharpness and accepted it without a second thought. As a grown-up, I wish I had been able to talk with her. For whatever reason, she felt free to be visibly discontented, and in contrast to the silence of the historical record, her will is fascinating. I cannot help but think of Ro when I read the diagnostic tests developed by doctors in the mid-twentieth century that were designed to assess women who exhibited ambivalence or a reluctance to become stay-at-home married mothers. Here are a few developed by W. S. Kroger, director of Psychosomatic Gynecology at Mount Sinai Hospital in Chicago: "Is the patient a cold, selfish, demanding person, or is she a warm, giving woman? . . . What is her motivation for becoming pregnant? . . . Could the absence of so-called 'motherliness' be due to environmental factors, permanent or temporary, and does this account for her sterility?" Ro's frustrations were inevitably complex, and easily dismissed as a personality trait rather than understood as a resentment of all the ways in which she was expected to act.

My mother convinced herself that it was not just possible but *right* to have a career in medicine and family—yet a professional working mother was remarkable enough even in the mid-1980s, when my brother was born, for *The New Zealand Woman's Weekly* (the equivalent of *US Weekly*) to run a story of the how-does-she-do-it variety about her. There was only one daycare facility in Auckland at the time. *One.* My mother fought like a demon to get both my brother and me enrolled in it.

My mother's seemingly unshakeable confidence rubbed off on me to the extent that when I told her of my low ovarian reserve levels, I was shocked by her own grief. She was also undone. She had, without ever telling me, saved many of my baby and toddler clothes, fully confident that one day, there would be a child or two to pass them on to. Now she sobbed over the phone. She had never explicitly expressed any expectation partly because she had assumed that she would never have to, that I would be quietly borne along by an inexorable current toward marriage and children without ever having to think too hard about it. And now I was cast up on a shore she did not recognize. I am sure she asked herself how it came to this: how she could have a daughter, half a world away, facing infertility in her midthirties.

My mother and father married in 1970, but it wasn't until 1980 that they had me, their first child. This delay was not really possible, my mother tells me, without oral contraceptives: in the intervening decade, they each finished graduate school, built a steel-hulled yacht, and sailed around the world together. When I ask my mother why they had me when they did, she says that it was time. When I ask my father, he says the pill failed. They are each adamant that they are right. I suspect there is a way in which they both are. I was conceived off the coast of Montevideo, and born in Bristol Harbor, in England. Eighteen months later, they sold the boat, and we all flew back to Aotearoa, to gardens and grandparents and blue skies. We bought a house in the suburbs. My brother was born. Our family settled in a rhythm of living that continued without disruption for the next fifteen years. My childhood now feels like a dream most days, another world.

For much of human history, our average life expectancy meant that women only had a small window of time within which to live as independent, unattached adults, without a child: a few years, if that. The distance between arrow and target was so small that any talk of delay was academic. My mother and I were able to draw out that first stage to a decade (for my mother), and fifteen years (for me). The distance became something tangible enough to manipulate. I only started to think about my fertility when I was making enough money to afford a child. My mother started thinking about hers when she realized she did not want to keep on sailing. We saw the horizon line of our days, and quietly changed our minds. I am very aware of our privilege, and the massed sea of women who either could not make a choice, or could not speak of the ones they did.

WHEN I WAS in my early thirties, I started to sense a kind of sphericity to my life, an inevitability to the shape of my existence. I felt it most clearly the days I wrote in cafes. There would be three, ten, fifteen people there. A few on laptops. Others sat together, talking. One might be dressed in nurse's scrubs. Another's father had just died. The third wore very large heart earrings. Sitting at the bar, a woman had a flock of starlings tattooed on her back. The fan might be turning, the Smiths playing. Out on the street, people would walk by in the soft light, inspecting their phones. Olives, water, wine. I could go to a different café, could come back here on another day and though the details—the food, customers, weather, and song—might be different, the feeling wouldn't have changed. I sensed some kind of hardening. You could call it a slowing. The plates of my experience were fusing together. I felt like I was living within my own horizon line, and hadn't departed from it for some time.

I could not stop thinking about Parmenides, a philosopher who lived in the fifth century BC in southern Italy, who was convinced that ontological pluralism—the belief that our existence is made up of many moments—was a misapprehension. Parmenides believed that our existence was one single, unchanging reality, in which the passing of time, space, and motion was an illusion. According to him, milk might sour, and loved ones might die, but the world was actually continuous, indivisible. Parmenides is slightly easier to understand if you imagine Italy in summer. There, the senses are sympathetic to an unchanging reality; the days have a rhythm, the pulse of a sleeping heart. Olive trees, sunshine, water; the sound of the wind in the leaves. Insects cry out, clinging to the bark. But I was in New York, and the one thing that seemed true here was that everything always seemed to be changing. Parmenides's arguments had long seemed completely crazy to me, until they didn't: as I sat in café after café, my life's repetitions took on a blurry heft. I started to understand how I might be living within a oneness of comprehension, where everything—even the things I had not yet experienced—was still inside the horizon line of my understanding. I could imagine myself here, at forty, at fifty, at sixty. My sense of predestination rose like sap in a plant.

Parmenides's lover was (reputedly) Zeno of Elea, another philosopher. You might recognize his name because Zeno's paradoxes are one of the few pieces of Greek philosophy that persist by name in popular culture today. The most commonly remembered one is about an arrow and a target. People remember the gist of it: a space—a football field, an arrow and target—and talk about moving from one end to the other in steps, each time dividing in half the remaining distance. You can move half of the way there, they say, and then half that, and so on and so forth, yet because you can halve the distance an infinite number of times, it should take an infinite amount of time to reach the target. That an arrow *does* hit its target suggested that those who thought the world was divisible were just plain wrong. Zeno's paradoxes were thought experiments designed to defend Parmenides: to both men, what we perceive as multiplicity is really a singularity wearing the mask of many.

We're so confident in our empiricism now that the scenario seems a pseudo-intellectual amusement rather than a real proposition, but Zeno was serious. His sense of indivisibility dogs the humanities in other ways, too: it is also a basis of spiritual belief. This might be why we remember Zeno's name. There is something about his thought experiments that is singular enough to name, a quality in his stories of division and non-attainment that we still find distinct. They are analogies for a thought process we seem to have a hard time explaining any other way. In some kind of asymptotic echo of his paradox, most people trail off before they get to the end of their retelling; they're confident of the bit about division, hazy about the conclusion. Our fuzziness about the paradox is part of the paradox now. His is the line of a song that everybody in a bar somehow knows to chant, in unison, even if they don't know the singer's name. "Oh! We're halfway there. Oh-oh!" It may be that Zeno's paradox persists because beyond his name, there is no single word that can accommodate that delicate sense of the finite and the infinite. Like oil and vinegar, if left alone long enough, they'll insist on separating. The paradox whisks them together. In those cafés, it *did* seem to take an infinity to walk to the bathroom.

One explanation for wanting a child—which now seems more persuasive to me than any biological clock or evolutionary urge—is that I was worried Parmenides was right in a way I couldn't understand, and I wanted to prove him wrong. After all, if I had a child, I would literally become divisible. It was a simple thought, but it would not go away. There was no way I would remain within this particular sphere of existence, no way I would remain in these cafés.

I would literally become something else. The lure of that division, that meiosis, grew. I wanted to experience a completely different scale of change. If there is any evolutionary or biological urge to procreate, I think it resides here, in my instinctive fascination with division.

A FEW YEARS AGO, on a visit back to New Zealand, my mother invited me to her choir's annual performance at the Auckland Town Hall. I'd never thought of my mother as someone who could carry a tune, but it was obviously a big deal for her, and so along I went.

The impression, upon entering the hall, was that the stage was stacked with women, row upon row, easily more than a hundred. On closer inspection, I could see men at the top, peppering the back rows. Most were Pākehā (white). My mother had told me about the conductor, about how all their songs were his arrangements of popular songs—but still it surprised me, when they opened their mouths to sing, that all of the songs were about love: love song after love song, some from my mother's generation, some from mine. These were not songs my mother listened to until they were arranged for her. There she was, standing two rows from the front, almost in the middle, watching the conductor with a hawk eye. Women were wearing bright colors: orange dresses, red dresses, skirts with flowers, dresses with sequins, dresses with birds of paradise on them or made from green saris. It looked like a school photo, but everyone was at least fifty years old and had their mouths open, their faces relaxed in concentration and joy.

I watched my mother singing about who had loved, and who had loved and lost. She was swaying from side to side, mimicking the conductor's hands with her head, nodding firmly on a downbeat, pulling up to hold a sustained note. I started to cry. I had not seen my mother ever sing about love. She had dealt with so much in the preceding two decades, and here she was on stage, in her sixties, willing to *sing*. They all were, these women, with the same no-nonsense look I associate with New Zealand women: short hair and sun spots, strong hands at their sides, harmonizing with each other, more than half a century of choices on stage. They had had children, or not had children, avoided falling pregnant and ended pregnancies, grieved children, partners, and parents, and now they were singing, caught in loops of lyric that suspended them through time, singing to their families about love. History's breath may have been on their neck, but they had also practiced inhaling and exhaling together. Here was an indivisible sphere: these women, stacked to the rafters, singing. *This could be me*, I thought, had I stayed here. I could be coming to choir practice. It was like seeing, all of a sudden, another path in the woods, an expedition had I not left home. All my posterity: these were women willing not to talk, but to sing.

5

. . .

SEEING

Sperm were first seen by Antonij van Leeuwenhoek, a Dutch milliner and city official, in Delft in 1677. He drew the "animalcules" he found, and described their proportions to William Brouncker, president of the Royal Society of London: "They were furnished with a thin tail about 5 or 6 times as long as the body, and very transparent and with the thickness of about one twenty-fifth that of the body." They swam like "a snake or an eel swimming in water," but in thicker material would "lash their tails at least 8 or 10 times before they could advance a hair's breadth." You can see exactly what he saw in the time it takes you to look up "sperm microscope" on YouTube. He's right. They radiate intensity, though they seem to be going nowhere fast.

It was a remarkable discovery. Leeuwenhoek had been experimenting for years with microscopes, grinding glass lenses and achieving ever greater powers of magnification, but up until 1674, his discoveries had been to magnify the already visible. Along with a group of microscope enthusiasts in Holland, France, and England, he had carefully documented the movement of sap, and the structure of muscle, bones, brains, spit, and cuticles. Some men diagrammed insects, others viperous dogfish. They wrote to each with their observations, and compared notes on microscope design. Leeuwenhoek also diligently sent his observations to the editor of *Philosophical Transactions*, Henry Oldenburg, in England, who encouraged him to continue, albeit with some reserve; Leeuwenhoek was considered an amateur, in a far-flung city. He didn't know English or Latin. There was also the awkward fact that the Dutch and the English were at war with one another. But it was obvious the milliner had drive and talent; he was secretive about his method of lens production, and the level of magnification he was able to achieve was remarkable enough for Robert Hooke, probably the most well-known naturalist working with the microscope in England at that time, to learn Dutch and translate Leeuwenhoek for Oldenburg.

Months before Leeuwenhoek had seen sperm, he had seen red blood cells, and had written to Oldenburg of these remarkable red globules. The editor hesitated to publish. It was a wild assertion, this world within a world, of living animals *inside* living animals. He asked Hooke to try to verify the experiments. It was only on Hooke's third try that the English scientist was finally able to also see microbes in water, and show them to other members of the Royal Society. Once they had all seen it for themselves, they conceded: Leeuwenhoek had discovered another world within their own.

Leeuwenhoek was likely an acquaintance of the painter Johannes Vermeer: Delft was a small town then, and the two were christened a fortnight apart in the same church. Precisely at the moment that Holland was becoming a colonial superpower, establishing trading stations as far-flung as Iran and Taiwan, both men inverted the ambition of their gaze, directing it inward. Vermeer also used lenses, purchasing a camera obscura. His emphasis on introspection in his paintings, on women reading, thinking, concentrating, is a strangely apt analogue for Leeuwenhoek's discovery of a world within a world. The women in his paintings are lit by windows, often beside them, but they rarely look outside. They use the light for something else: to read, write, sew. (One of the reasons Vermeer's work remains compelling is how interested he is in painting a woman thinking and working.) Leeuwenhoek's letters to Oldenburg are unrepentantly interested in a subject that he knows concerns very few. He is interested in what his peers think, not what the world does. It is a quasi-domestic scale of scientific discovery: men, separated by continents, writing to each other of their findings. Others who were sympathetically minded brought Leeuwenhoek curiosities. (It was a medical school student from Leiden who provided Leeuwenhoek with the sperm sample.) It is almost a painting: here are slides of blood, spit, and semen. Here are grasses, picked from the edge of town. The corpses of small animals are piled in the yard. All these discoveries, set among life itself: through the window, the cry of a baby who won't stop crying, who is teething. And here is Leeuwenhoek, sitting at his desk, looking into his microscope, drawing what he sees.

THE HUMAN EGG was not seen for another 150 years. This is despite the fact that it is the largest cell in the body, and the only one that can be seen with the naked eye. It is as big as the period at the end of this sentence.

In the history of human knowledge, this event seems almost comically out of place. By 1827, Michael Faraday had already developed the first rudimentary electric motor. That year, Joseph Niépce made the first modern photograph. The telegraph was barely a decade away. The gas light had been invented.

There were people who had tried looking before. In 1672—five years before Leeuwenhoek saw sperm—the Dutch anatomist Regnier de Graaf dissected a number of female rabbits a few days after they had mated. When cutting into the ovary, he noticed a number of spherical structures inside that had reddened and ruptured. He concluded that these might be eggs.

The idea that a mammal might grow from an egg had been at least a theoretical possibility since the seventeenth century, when the English physician William Harvey coined the phrase *ex ovo omnia* ("everything comes from an egg"), but it was one thing to idly consider the consistency of a thought, and another to actually look for an egg inside a woman. Numerous attempts were probably made by men dissecting female human corpses, but unless the woman was ovulating right when she died, the egg would likely be encased in the follicle, and not visible in the fallopian tubes. (Even if she had ovulated, a white speck would've been difficult to spot among the other organs as they decomposed.) This was de Graaf's mistake; he mistook the rabbit follicles for the egg itself. He knew that something was wrong; by his calculations, the egg should have been far smaller than the follicles he found—but he could never square the discrepancy. He died a year later.

In a similar experiment but more than a century later, in Dorpat, Russia, the Estonian-born scientist Karl Ernst von Baer noticed, when visiting a colleague, that their family dog was in heat. They decided to kill her and look for her eggs. In his account, he described opening the ovaries and piercing the follicles with a knife. Inside, there was a "minuscule and well-developed yellow sphere of yolk...."

It was such a rare sight—an egg that actually looked like an egg—that he "shrank back as if struck by lightning."

Von Baer must've continued his efforts with humans, because in 1827 he published "On the Genesis of the Ovum of Mammals and of Man," and drew the first visual representation of a human egg. The plate that concludes the book includes twenty or so details from the reproductive systems of animals, including dogs, porpoises, rabbits, monkeys, birds, mollusks, frogs, salamanders, lizards, insects, crayfish, and spiders. The human egg is a dot, a tiny planet in an esoteric cosmology of animal fertility; if you didn't read the illustrative key carefully enough, you would hardly know it existed.

Von Baer didn't really account for his circumspection. Though he described his dissections of dogs in detail, the same sense of narrative occasion wasn't granted to the human ovum. In his book, he noted he had dissected two different women: one, a prostitute, and the second, a young girl who had committed suicide, and who was found to be pregnant. In both cases, he wrote, no eggs were found—which left his discovery of the human egg unexplained. Indeed, his silence about this moment of discovery is so marked that one suspects the story was far more morally complicated than he could acknowledge. At the time, corpses available for dissection tended to be people convicted of various crimes. Von Baer couldn't resist including his discovery, hiding in plain sight, but his explanation of the matter is remarkably far from Leeuwenhoek's lengthy correspondence and Hooke's replications of the experiment for the entire Royal Society, the oldest national scientific institution in the world. Von Baer's egg slipped into history with no peer review, no announcement, barely a narrative.

The differing weight given to the visual discovery of sperm and ovum is striking, but not surprising. In the seventeenth century, the popular preformist view of reproduction was that organisms developed from miniature versions of themselves. In 1694, the microscopist Nicolaas Hartsoeker drew a tiny person crouched inside a sperm, curled up in an embryonic position, as some researchers had claimed to see. His drawings resemble William Blake's. He called it a homunculus. The French priest and philosopher Nicolas Malebranche took it a step further, suggesting that each embryo contained an even smaller embryo, which contained a smaller one and so on and so forth: all of human history nested inside itself like a set of matryoshka dolls—which had been created, at one point in time, by God. (The idea is not so outré as it sounds; it is strikingly similar to some theories of reincarnation. It seems likely that Parmenides, had he lived in the seventeenth century, would've been a preformist.) A preformist rationale was a natural attempt to account for the soul—how on earth could a soul *develop*? Leeuwenhoek was highly dismissive of Hartsoeker's homunculus and thought the claim a hoax, but he still assumed that it was sperm and sperm alone that was responsible for creating human life. He thought the sperm he'd seen under his microscope were simply parasites of some kind, and the *surrounding* liquid was responsible for reproduction. In it, he wrote, he saw a large variety of other kinds of microscopic vessels, and thought they were the beginning of the human vascular system. (It should go without saying that no subsequent observer was able to replicate that result.) Even if these men accepted the likelihood of an egg existing, they followed the Aristotelian line that semen gave women's "matter" form. Most monotheistic religions considered semen the primary component in creation too.

More than a millennium before, Aristotle had observed fetal development in chickens by poking holes in eggs and observing the growing chicken fetuses. He saw how they gradually acquired a beating heart, bones, and feathers. Experiments like these led to an epigenetic school of thought about reproductive development—that life is created by a developing series of parts that grow increasingly differentiated over time—which also held sway in the seventeenth century. It wasn't an easy sell for a long time, largely because it wasn't until the nineteenth century that an adequate explanation developed for how small simple things could possibly grow to become so complex. Cell theory showed that cell division, a mechanism for growth, might begin to account for the transformative energy needed to create human life. But for Leeuwenhoek and others, working more than a century before that realization, it appeared that preformist and epigenetic schools were so diametrically opposed, so perfectly counterfactual to each other, that they exerted some kind of intrinsic magnetism; it was hard to be an epigeneticist without coming up against some hard preformist questions, and vice versa. Not incidentally, these positions are echoed in current abortion debates. Thus Leeuwenhoek, who described sperm so accurately, misidentified their purpose so quickly.

AT SOME POINT you might wonder: Does it really matter to see inside? Is it important to "discover" something so innate? Does it make a difference who saw it first? We did quite well for ourselves as a species for hundreds of thousands of years without seeing any of this. Western medicine, with its focus on sight, its anxiety about proof, is hardly the only way to know a body.

In the 1960s—right as the pill was legalized, and at the height of the post–World War II baby boom—a number of books and magazines published detailed color photographs of fetuses. The most famous were Lennart Nilsson's photographs for *Life* magazine in 1965, which you've probably seen without knowing who took them. You can trace the developing capillaries in the legs, as distinct as the veins on a tree leaf, the caul like tissue paper, the fine hairs on the forehead. The fetuses' anatomical strangeness is not emphasized; Nilsson's images demonstrate how *like* an infant a fetus can be. Within days, the magazine's entire print run of 8 million copies had sold out. In other words: at precisely the time when women sought more choice, their sense of what that choice amounted to was also changing.

Nilsson was not alone; many other books sought to emphasize the fetus's personhood. Geraldine Flanagan's *The First Nine Months of Life* (1962) is particularly noteworthy because it carefully explains the cellular development of an embryo and fetus, all the while attributing complex human emotion to the photos: for instance, a fetus is "sucking its thumb" or "crying." She wrote that every baby has a "lie," a favorite position for sleep, now and later, and included images of a fetus, legs bent open like a frog's, and another curled up on its side. She dismissed the notion that fetuses had gills or tails at one point, and showed a number of arresting images of fetal hands at different stages of development in weeks 5, 6, 7, and 8 (when they rapidly develop from buds to distinct fingers), and finally in the third month. She also continually stressed how early major organs and bodily systems developed, noting, for instance, how an embryo's heart begins to beat when it's less than a month old.

Flanagan also included, on four pages, a series of stills from movies of fetuses at varying ages (between 7 and 12 weeks). She noted that these fetuses had been stroked with a fine hair and their reflexes documented. They were given a small metal rod to grasp. In some of these images, the adult human hand was clearly visible, offering scale but also the clear sense of how beautifully miniaturized the fetus was, how exact and precise its construction. In the seventh week, she noted, when the upper lip is stroked, "the back muscles contract and the arms move back." It was obvious she wanted her readers to bond with these images, the underlying assumption being that when you can perceive the profile of a face—eyes, brow, mouth—or the outline of a body, you are more likely to understand that the fetus inside is an individual in their own right. The book quietly relied on the expectation that to see an object, to uncover the normally hidden, would make it seem more real. It was a rear-guard preformist interpretation of embryonic and fetal development, pronatalist and anti-abortion, though the accompanying text did not acknowledge this. Ian Donald, the British surgeon who developed ultrasound, was widely known to use ultrasound to persuade women *not* to have an abortion.

Flanagan and Nilsson did not specify the more uncomfortable fact that the fetuses and embryos in their books were all—by virtue of their being photographed—dead or dying. Flanagan used images from the Carnegie Institution of Washington's collection. (A former director of the institution, George W. Corner, wrote the foreword, and emphasized the book's scientific accuracy as well as its esthetic appeal; the young mother would "gain from these pages an enhanced sense of the dignity and essential beauty of her experience.") Flanagan also did not mention that the stills of fetal movement she used were from a series of experiments carried out between the 1930s and 1960s by neuroanatomist Davenport Hooker at the University of Pittsburgh. Hooker studied the nervous system of fetuses in their final minutes of life. The embryos came to the lab directly from the operating room, and were immediately immersed in saline solution warmed to 90 degrees Fahrenheit. Hooker had a window of between 7 and 10 minutes for embryos and 20 minutes for older fetuses before they asphyxiated. He ended up observing 149 fetuses, regularly using a horsehair brush to elicit and measure a physical reaction, and filmed the results, producing the silent film *Early Fetal Human Activity* (1952). You can watch it on the internet. It is in black and white, and comes with extensive scientific intertitles. We see six fetuses, each tiny, glowing white against the darkness. When stroked with a single hair, they react the way we do in sleep—instinctively, with a short and sharp movement. As the film progresses, the fetuses increase in size. Their legs and hands twitch; their head jerks away from the feather or rod.

One measure of the effect these images have had on our sense of what is inside us is how difficult they are to watch. The fetuses' slenderness is pronounced. Hooker was not the only scientist to experiment on still-living fetuses. Herbert Evens used to inject tiny fetal hearts with india ink to show the "multitudinous vascular channels." Others preferred to inject fetuses with fixative while still alive, thinking it produced finer specimens. We have learned to humanize fetuses in a way that would have been deeply unfamiliar to women who could not look inside themselves even two hundred years ago. Saint Augustine argued that "ensoulment" happened when a woman experienced "quickening," which was her sensation of the fetus inside (usually at four to five months). This was the official position of the Catholic Church until the nineteenth century (though there were a few early Christian writers who argued that early abortion was infanticide). Other theories mark the arrival of a soul as being at the time of birth, or the time the child first laughs. Many cultures have told stories about women who've given birth to nonhuman things, among them gold and jewelry, monkeys, fish stomachs, and kangaroos. But by now, it is difficult for any woman born in the late twentieth or early twenty-first century to *not* think of fetal photographs and ultrasounds when she thinks of life inside her. (It is also not a practice confined to wealthy nations: ultrasound imaging and stills are extremely popular in developing countries too.) The egg may have taken centuries to see, but the embryo is now everywhere.

It is not "just" looking, either. From the 1970s on, a wave of feminist scholarship began to point out the ways in which ultrasound technology purported to offer a "verifiable" image that was actually very hard for a woman to decipher herself. Even with improvements in image quality since the 1950s, a patient still had a hard time recognizing much beyond the curve of the fetal skull. Her uterus may have become the visible object, but she could not decipher her own meaning: she had ceded interpretive power to the doctor or sonographer, waiting anxiously for them to speak, to explain what it is they can see—that is the ear, that is the hand, that is the feet. In her landmark study of women undergoing sonography, the anthropologist Lisa M. Mitchell paused to consider what it actually meant when women said they "saw" their baby during an ultrasound. Her conclusion was that their seeing was actually listening to the sonographer's interpretation, to being told what the whites of the image (bone) and blacks (liquid) were: once again, sound understood as sight. In follow-up interviews, women's descriptions closely paralleled the sonographer's descriptions. We have come a long way from Leeuwenhoek's sperm or von Baer's drawing of an egg, and yet we remain uncertain about what it is, exactly, we are seeing, all the while convinced that it is a laudable effort to try.

Our bodies have no interest in our aesthetic conception of ourselves. The uterus—despite how it is drawn—is not actually a hollow-looking vase of flesh. It is a piece of flesh approximately 3 cm in length, its walls pressing against each other. But our minds—our minds have *every* interest in our aesthetic conceptions of our bodies, and it is a persistent enough habit across human history to elevate sight, and to understand it as a direct analogue for knowledge, to suspect that epistemologies of vision derive their value *through* a process of detachment, of insisting upon some kind of separation precisely when there is none.

When I was younger, I didn't really see the point of a Cartesian separation; it never resonated with my own experience of mind and body, which appeared absolutely dependent on one another: what the body went through (running, eating, sex) appeared to largely determine the thoughts a mind could have, and vice versa. If we thought of our brains as a source of abstraction, it seemed to me a habit of mind that probably had an evolutionary function. But I am starting to take the persistent tic of mind that conceives of itself as separate from the body more seriously. It has to do, in part, with my infertility: I was confronted by how much I didn't know my own body, know what was going on inside of it.

Even now, the gap still feels wide and vast. The public record and the public body have very rarely been one and the same. Our identification of our own living form extends far beyond ourselves,

throughout the natural world, from life to death and back again—
tracing a kind of elliptical planetary orbit around the actual sense of
what it feels for us to be inside ourselves. We dance around the egg
and the embryo. They remain, in some sense, as abstract as language,
even though they are the primary building blocks of our being.

6

. . .

HE SAID/HE SAID

In 1980, Patrick Steptoe and Robert Edwards published *A Matter of Life*, their account of producing the world's first IVF baby, Louise Brown. They took turns writing chapters, their narratives intertwining, a kind of he said/he said of collegial scientific harmony. They relied on dates and details, on what appeared (at least in the first half of the book) to be an unadorned storytelling.

They began with their separate beginnings. Steptoe was the older man; he graduated from St. George's Hospital Medical School in London in 1939, seven years after the publication of Huxley's *Brave New World*, and joined the Royal Navy Volunteer Reserve as a surgeon. After World War II he resumed his medical training, specializing in obstetrics, partly as a result of his experience in the navy and as a prisoner of war in Italy, where he had seen enough pain and suffering. It was "refreshing," he wrote, "to deliver a healthy baby to a delighted woman!" It wasn't just the war that pushed him in this direction, either; it had been impressed upon him from childhood that it was a good thing to do good for pregnant women. He was named after the doctor who delivered him, and his mother founded the local Mothers' Union and Infant Welfare Clinic in his town, Witney. He grieved the consequences of poor medical care. One of the most moving parts of *A Matter of Life* is his description of a woman who had been admitted to a London hospital after a botched illegal abortion. She developed tetanus, beginning with lockjaw and proceeding to full-body rigidity. In general, Steptoe was not in the habit of providing lingering descriptive detail in his book, but he took the time to describe her pain and suffering: "The involvement of her facial muscles caused her to grin grotesquely. Terrible spasms would begin as the result of the slightest stimuli—a jarring of her bed, a draught of cold air, a noise of any kind, a light switched on in the corridor when the door opened. At her post mortem I felt angry before her body on the slab . . . the pale face at last at rest, the striking red hair—angry as I observed the pathologist demonstrate how her abortion had been cruelly botched." This could be viewed as voyeuristic, but I think Steptoe would've said it was also one way to acknowledge and name the tragedy of her death. This was a different kind of suffering than what he'd encountered in the war; senseless, but preventable.

In London it was virtually impossible to find a specialist's position; the competition was just too fierce. Steptoe decided to travel to the industrial north, and took up a position in Oldham Hospital, near Manchester. It was, symbolically and literally, a move to the provinces, yet there were advantages. Steptoe was isolated from his peers, but he also had a huge amount of freedom and considerable responsibility. The list of women in Oldham waiting for surgery on the NHS was thousands long. The degree of suffering was marked. "I had never seen women with such enormous tumours, such degrees of uterine prolapse," he wrote. He threw himself into the job. The only other obstetrician was Catholic, and so, in a catchment area of 300,000 people, Steptoe was responsible for all abortions and sterilizations.

In 1951, the same year Steptoe began working in Oldham (at thirty-eight), Edwards was starting his PhD in embryology at the University of Edinburgh. This was not a particularly well-thought-out career plan: Edwards first studied agriculture as an undergraduate, decided that seeds bored him, and so in his final year moved on to zoology and animal seeds. The shift helped clarify his interests, but it was too late for his grades; he graduated with indifferent results, and out of desperation, followed a friend to Edinburgh University. Like Steptoe, Edwards was always careful to emphasize the ways in which chance and circumstance begat his sense of experimentation, but he was also (in his words) the "competitive second son of a working-class family." He happened to attend a lecture by Alan Beatty, who had essentially carried out the process of IVF (and embryo transfer) with a mouse: he had taken an egg from one mouse, fertilized it, then transferred it to the uterus of another mouse, whereupon it had successfully implanted. Beatty agreed to supervise Edwards for his PhD, and Edwards threw himself into the production of haploid mouse embryos, which were embryos that lacked a full set of forty chromosomes (useful in identifying gene expression). Mice breed prodigiously when left to their own devices, but doing the job for them was much harder. Edwards had to irradiate the spermatozoa, which deactivated certain chromosomes; identify when the mice were in estrus (day or night); and grow the embryo in a suitable medium. The "next-ness" in Edwards's narrative, the way in which each step is presented as logical, even simple, occasionally occludes the sheer amount of work involved, which was painstaking, repetitive, and far from abstract. The labor involved in embryology was also a craft that took years to refine. One developed a physical intuition for materials. In four months, Edwards was only able to produce two haploid embryos. It took a year before he was producing embryos with any regularity.

Steptoe and Edwards weren't the first to think about IVF with mammalian eggs. Some efforts were well documented, particularly by Walter Heape, who in 1890 transferred rabbit embryos from one female to another. In *A Matter of Life*, Edwards also notes that Gregory Pincus in America—co-inventor of the combined oral contraceptive pill—carried out a number of experiments with rabbits in the 1930s, including in vitro fertilization and parthenogenesis. These experiments were later challenged; Pincus did not provide enough documentation, and his clinical results couldn't be replicated. A similar quandary beset John Rock and Miriam Menkin, who in 1944 extracted a woman's egg, bathed it in sperm, and reported a successful fertilization. Critics insisted that because it had not been successfully implanted, there was no way of telling whether the egg's cleavage was actually fertilization or reflex cell division.

In their book, Edwards and Steptoe documented the efforts of Heape, Pincus, Rock, and Menkin. Where they fell silent is the case of Landrum Brewer Shettles, who in the 1950s, working out of Columbia Presbyterian Medical Center in New York City, recreated Rock and Menkin's experiments. Shettles collected a large number of immature oocytes from women undergoing gynecological surgery at Columbia and fertilized them with his own sperm. These women were almost certainly unaware that in the course of a hysterectomy or surgical treatment of polycystic ovarian syndrome (which, at that point, involved the removal of a part of the ovary), their eggs were being taken and fertilized by Shettles. When asked by an interviewer later how he obtained the eggs, Shettles replied, "Most of them I just poached." He photographed hundreds of fertilized eggs, later publishing a visual encyclopedia, *Ovum Humanum*, in 1960, but he barely kept any written record of the date, circumstances, or experimental methods he used. Later, he claimed that in 1962 he achieved a successful IVF transfer of a fertilized embryo into another woman's uterus (she was due for a hysterectomy a week later, and gave her consent to see if it would successfully implant, which it did), but Shettles kept absolutely no record of any of this work, and couldn't even recall the woman's name. Given the scientific prestige that would've been accorded to Shettles if he succeeded, his claim appears to have been either false or evidence of a pathologically self-defeating personality.

He wasn't alone: in 1961, an Italian scientist named Daniele Petrucci claimed he had created forty human embryos through IVF, and said he had grown one of them in the laboratory for nearly a month. He claimed that it had developed a heartbeat, and was deformed. Petrucci went on to work in the Soviet Union, at the Institute of Experimental Biology in Moscow, developing artificial wombs. His team later claimed to have cultivated 250 embryos there, including one fetus for six months. Before it died, they said, it weighed one pound two ounces (about half the size that would usually be expected at that gestational age). It is very hard to understand how this was possible then, as it has not been replicated since, and no "proof" was forthcoming. Fairly regularly in these decades, doctors reported to the media extraordinary achievements in reproductive technologies that were never verified, and never published in peer-reviewed journals. One of the most famous cases was the book *In His Image*, in which David M. Rorvik, a nonfiction writer (and past collaborator with Shettles) claimed he had cloned another human being on an island in the South Pacific. The account sounded like a novel: Rorvik extracted eggs from an indigenous woman on the unnamed island, and managed to implant a body cell nucleus from a secretive sixty-five-year-old millionaire called Max into the cytoplasm of a human ovum. This embryo, in turn, was implanted into a woman called Sparrow. The book sold spectacularly, but Rorvik was later successfully sued by a British scientist called Derek Bromhall for plagiarizing part of his doctoral thesis.

Cases like Petrucci and Rorvik were easy to dismiss, but Edwards couldn't have missed how similar some of Shetttles's methods were to his own. Edwards also relied on his research connections to obtain tissue from a hospital setting, first asking the gynecologist who delivered his daughter to give him excised pieces of ovarian tissue which she removed during her various surgeries. He literally stood in the back of the operating theatre, gloved and masked, empty dish in hand. In 1963 (one year after Shettles), Edwards also tried to fertilize three ova with his own semen. He observed one almost-fertilization: a sperm had made its way partly through the zona pellucida, but not the whole way inside. He knew the results wouldn't count for much, but couldn't help but try, just to see what would happen. Just as with Shettles, it seems very unlikely those women would've given their consent to Edwards. (He does not mention it in the book.) Other doctors at Cambridge Hospital disliked his requests for ovarian tissue. "Perhaps I explained myself badly, or was too enthusiastic," he wrote, "or the issues of fertilization carried a more emotional charge than I realized." It is a somewhat remarkable understatement. Edwards was so driven by the idea of fertilization outside the body, and so comfortable with creating mouse embryos *en masse*, that he seems to have underestimated the difference in kind in creating human embryos.

Implicitly, where he distinguishes himself from Shettles in the narrative is his emphasis on experimental design and verifiable results. He was willing to document his failures. During a visit to Johns Hopkins University for six weeks in 1965, he wanted to work out a way to expose sperm to the female reproductive tract. (At that point, it was believed that the sperm were "activated" by some kind of chemical signal from the vagina, cervix, or fallopian tubes that then allowed them to penetrate an egg.) Edwards took a number of approaches. He tried fertilizing eggs with sperm that had been in a cervix (collecting them just after patients had sex). Then he tried mimicking the conditions of the cervix by adding small pieces of uterus or fallopian tube to the culture in which he'd placed egg and sperm. He also tried putting human eggs and sperm inside the fallopian tubes of a rabbit. Then he tried the fallopian tubes of rhesus monkeys. Nothing worked. The following summer, he upped the ante, creating small cages with porous walls and filling them with sperm. He inserted these chambers in the uteruses of female volunteers and left them overnight: uterine secretions could pass through the walls, but sperm couldn't leave. He took this sperm, and tried to fertilize eggs in dishes. That didn't work either.

One gains the impression—borne out by other colleagues and biographers—that Edwards was a restless, creative, and deeply ambitious man, willing to change direction in order to keep up some kind of research momentum. Until the mid-1960s, Edwards was pursuing several lines of research in animal embryos and hadn't settled on human infertility as a focus. His own self-assessment of the risks he took seems to be tempered, at least in his memoir, by how much of a family man he was at the time; during these decades of experimentation, he also raised five daughters with the geneticist Ruth Edwards (née Rutherford, the granddaughter of Ernest). Life in the suburbs of Cambridge inevitably created an easy origin story for the idea of IVF: a visit from a childless couple, and Edwards's rumination on their loss. It was also an account that reframed his ambition. Science could be a means to a widely sanctioned end: more babies, more families, and supposedly, more happiness.

In 1967, browsing through the latest medical journals, Edwards came across a description of a new surgical technique called laparoscopy. The method enables exploring the inside of an abdomen without making a large incision: instead, the laparoscope may be inserted through the umbilicus. Generally understood today as pinhole surgery, it greatly minimizes the chances of complication and infection. The article's writer, Patrick Steptoe, described collecting sperm from the fallopian tubes as if it were no big thing. This was precisely what Edwards needed—a way to extract a fully mature egg without excising tissue, and to gather sperm that had been exposed to the female reproductive system. Edwards rang Steptoe immediately—but then got cold feet. If they were to collaborate, it would involve a regular 165-mile commute between Cambridge and Oldham that would take hours on winding roads. They would have to persuade a woman entering the hospital for a hysterectomy to have sex with her husband before the operation, so that Steptoe could gather both sperm in the fallopian tubes and her eggs at the same time. Edwards would have very little notice and would need to begin driving immediately. There was no embryology lab in Oldham, so they would need to build one. The hurdles were so considerable that it wasn't until a chance encounter in London six months later, at the Royal Society of Medicine, that Edwards and Steptoe met face to face, sized each other up, and decided that it was worth a try.

By then, Steptoe had been working in Oldham for almost thirty years, and Edwards in Cambridge for fifteen. They were already well into their careers. Part of their success together would come from an almost military distribution of responsibility: Steptoe would deal with the patients and the surgery, Edwards with the lab. They hired a lab assistant, Jean Purdy, who had been a nurse, who would work as a lab technician for them, monitoring eggs and, hopefully, embryos. Purdy relocated to Oldham, they assembled a basic lab in a spare room at Oldham Hospital, and they began to work together. Almost immediately, they experienced considerable success: in a new kind of culture medium created by Barry Bavister, one of Edwards's former students, the eggs Steptoe removed from women were fertilized over and over again, without having to expose the sperm to uterine secretions. The belief that female fluids were required to "prepare" sperm for fertilization turned out to not be true after all—and with it, many of Edwards's earlier experiments in the 1960s with chambers and pieces of uterus in culture could be put to rest. Steptoe, Edwards, and Purdy began to regularly document embryos that were between one and three days old. They photographed the elegant division: one into two cells, two into four, four into eight, each as distinct as a petal, arranged in the shape of a flower. Within two years of meeting each other, they were able to publish a paper in *Nature* in 1969 that documented the fertilization of a human egg outside the womb that was not some kind of parthenogenesis (as was claimed about Rock and Menkin's experiment).

It was inevitable that the media would seize on this announcement. The image of a baby in a bottle was well established in dystopian literature. Huxley's descriptions of the cloning process in *Brave New World* were perhaps most well-known, particularly his image of a warehouse of babies in bottles: "the bulging flanks" of glass bottles in receding rows, arranged in tiers, "visible and crimson, like the darkness of closed eyes on a summer's afternoon." The malign innocence of this description is remarkable. As many writers, including Huxley, had deliberately smudged the distinction between science fiction and science, the public was primed to imagine the implications of outsourcing conception. Huxley's sense of consequence was also particularly well mapped out to play with class anxieties in Britain. In *Brave New World*, the embryos are cloned, then subjected to differing rates of hormones, vibration, and temperature changes in order to produce classes of human: those suited to hard labor, or those who love the tropics. Seventy percent of all female fetuses are rendered sterile with testosterone. Decanted from their bottles, the children are then brought up in mass-education facilities. Huxley taught biology at Eton, a boarding school—where he had the writer George Orwell as a student—and was quite aware of the construction of class privilege, and the effects of removing children from their families. Biological homogeneity begets social control. At the beginning of *Brave New World*, the reader tours a dormitory of sixty young boys and girls, all asleep, listening to an incessant monologue in a soft voice over the speakers: "Oh no, I *don't* want to play with Delta children. And Epsilons are still worse. They're too stupid to be able to read and write. Besides, they wear black, which is such a beastly color. I'm so glad I'm a Beta." The soft burr of microdistinction isn't futuristic at all. A group of working-class babies are presented with flowers, which then explode. These children will grow up hating the countryside, which, as the Director of the Central London Hatchery and Conditioning Centre concludes, suits everyone rather well. No one raised in the hatchery, the Director notes, knows what a family is, or that people once had their own, individual biological mother. This kind of escalation was so expertly written that, decades later, journalists couldn't resist going there. On reading Steptoe and Edwards's research, William Breckon in the *Times* feared a kind of breeding arms race, with each country working to produce a group of hyperintelligent humans. He wrote: "Ultimately we could have the know-how to breed these groups of human beings—called 'clones' after the Greek word for a throng— to produce a cohort of super-astronauts or dustmen, soldiers or senators, each with identical physical and mental characteristics most suited to do the job they have to do." Other headlines included "Doctors Start Baby Outside the Womb" (*The Guardian*), "Babies Storm Growing" (*Daily Express*), and "Ban the Test Tube Baby" (*The Sun*). Nearly all these articles were negative and/or inaccurate.

I suspect Edwards and Steptoe dismissed these concerns because they were hyperbolic, and because scaremongering headlines had no bearing on what they were actually able to do. The two men knew how far away they were from successfully implanting an embryo, let alone cloning one. The difference between dystopian rhetoric and the reality of a patient, sitting in a consultation room, unable to concentrate on anything but their desire to be a parent, was so distinct that Edwards and Steptoe barely bothered to explain themselves. They thought anyone actually confronted with the prospect of infertility would very quickly re-categorize the science, moving it from a reordering of the reproductive firmament to a basic clinical therapy. They didn't see it as their job to lead others to this conclusion.

They also had a different scale by which to measure their progress. One summer evening in 1970, Jean Purdy rang Edwards in Cambridge. She was in Oldham, observing a number of human embryos growing in culture that were now four days old. "Something is happening," she said. "Things I've not seen before." Edwards drove through the night to see them. To their knowledge, it was the first time that anyone had been able to document this next stage of embryo development, in which the outer wall appeared to solidify, and internal divisions between each cell softened and disappeared. The number of cells increased to between eighty and one hundred. The center of the sphere seemed to fill with liquid, and the cell growth at its edges became immensely complicated. The embryo, now called a blastocyst, resembled a bomb crater: smoothness in the middle, rubble around the rim. Visually speaking, the difference between a four-day embryo and a blastocyst was as big as the distance between a single violin and a symphony orchestra.

This is one of the few moments in *A Matter of Life* where you can hear the awe in Edwards's voice. (It is also the only place where he uses the word *beautiful* frequently): "It was an unbelievable sight: four beautiful human blastocysts, round spheres of cells filled with fluid, with their two types of cell—one thin and delicate, on the surface of each sphere, destined to turn into the placenta, which would nourish the foetus throughout the nine months' gestation; the other a beautiful disc of foetal cells, the beginning of the foetus as it started its journey towards life. Light, transparent, floating, expanding slightly, but still smaller than a pinpoint: there they were, four excellent blastocysts. The intrinsic beauty of it!" It is a moment

Edwards cannot help but repeatedly aestheticize. The blastocyst was so much more beautiful than any bottle on a conveyor belt. *This* was what was truly visible.

In 1971, Edwards and Steptoe decided to start implanting fertilized embryos in women. There were many in the scientific community—not just the media—who thought it foolhardy, ethically wrong, and dangerous. The pair were denied funding by the Medical Research Council, and scientific luminaries weighed in in very public ways: James Watson, who had mapped the structure of DNA, declared that Edwards and Steptoe were risking infanticide. Various studies hinted at genetic mutation; one paper, published in the early 1970s, described mice born through IVF with extremely small eyes. The implication was that the IVF process had genetically affected the mice's DNA. The author of the paper later realized his results were wrong, and that the mice's eyes were small because of that particular strain of mouse, not because of the technique—but the damage had been done. Many scientists didn't understand why Edwards and Steptoe couldn't first experiment on primates as a stepping stone between small mammals like mice, rats, and rabbits and humans, not realizing that in other primates the cervical canal was more convoluted, and that embryo transfers would be exponentially more complicated. In Edwards's view, embryos that were one to three days old were small, but extremely resistant to stress. They had, as he wrote, "the innate capacity to reorder and reform, to overcome the effects of drugs, X-rays, and other seemingly noxious agents that scientists have exposed them to." (That innate capacity would later become controversial for other reasons.) In Edwards's eyes, the embryo either died or grew normally. There wasn't much in between. He figured it would be the same for humans. His instinct and Steptoe's experience led the two men to push ahead with a speed that scared others.

There were incidents that showed cause for alarm. In 1973—unbeknownst to Edwards and Steptoe—a woman called Doris Del-Zio arrived at New York Hospital with her husband, John. They were there because their doctor, William Sweeney, who had operated on her for blocked fallopian tubes twice before, was willing to attempt to surgically remove her eggs via laparoscopy, fertilize them in a test tube, then reimplant them. Sweeney knew Landrum Shettles up at Columbia, and had proposed they collaborate: Sweeney would remove the ova, and Shettles would fertilize them and after two days, transfer them back into her uterus. Doris Del-Zio signed consent forms. The eggs would have to be taken by cab from one hospital to the other, so after Sweeney aspirated a vial of follicular fluid, and while Doris was recovering, her husband hailed a cab, with her eggs literally in hand. He did not think twice that he was met at the door of the hospital by Shettles rather than shown to his office, nor that he was sent to the men's bathroom to obtain a semen sample. Shettles simply took the two test tubes from him in the lobby, and said he'd be in touch. In a tissue-culture lab on the sixteenth floor (which did not belong to him), Shettles mixed the test tubes together, sealed it, and placed it inside an incubator which kept the sample at a temperature of 98 degrees Fahrenheit. He told the woman whose lab it actually was—Dominique Toran-Allerand—what he was doing, and she was horrified. She later said the sample "resembled a frothy chocolate milkshake" and believed that inserting it into a woman's uterus would lead to infection. She alerted her supervisor, who called Raymond Vande Wiele, the department's chairman. It was highly unlikely there had been any fertilization (the incubator didn't monitor carbon dioxide concentration, which is necessary for fertilization, and the type of black test tube stopper Shettles was using was known to emit fumes and inhibit cell division). Even if there was, the procedure was halted the next morning when the test tube was removed from the incubator without Shettles's knowledge and placed on Vande Wiele's desk.

Vande Wiele had intervened because he was worried that the experiment would jeopardize millions of dollars of funding from the government: Columbia had signed a code of behavior issued by the US Department of Health, Education, and Welfare that was expected to apply to all research conducted under federal grants. The Del-Zios hadn't paid for Shettles to fertilize her eggs, and his salary was, in part, paid by federal funding. Vande Wiele had protected Shettles in the past—he hadn't fired him, when others had called for that— but he was tired of Shettles's grandstanding. In 1971, *Look* magazine had prominently featured Shettles and his predictions. The title of the article was "Taking Life in Our Own Hands—A Historic Step: The Test-Tube Baby Is Coming." The cover was of a distinctly human fetus, perhaps 13 weeks old, in its amniotic sac, resting on the palm of Shettles's hand. The article made much of a recent study in which a 7-week embryo was kept alive for several hours in an oxygenated saline solution after being surgically removed from the uterus. This focus recapitulated the old fantasy of ectogenesis, and conflated the petri dish with the artificial womb. Shettles was confirming the worst of the media's speculation, rather than correcting it. Vande Wiele's worry about the hospital's liability was confirmed: the Del-Zios later sued Raymond Vande Wiele, Columbia University, and Presbyterian Hospital for the "intentional infliction of emotional distress," and sought $1.5 million in damages. Doris Del-Zio wasn't informed of the news that her eggs had not fertilized until more than twenty-four hours later, well after Shettles met with Vande Wiele. The news sent her into a deep depression that didn't lift for years. The month her child would have been born, she woke from a faint in a Florida department store, her arms full of baby clothes.

Doris Del-Zio's grief, documented in her lawsuit (they were awarded $50,000 for distress), is one of the few descriptions of how women dealt with the vertiginous possibility of IVF in the 1970s, one of the only moments when it is not he said/he said, but what *she* said. It was not an incident acknowledged by Edwards or Steptoe in their own book. In *A Matter of Life*, Edwards and Steptoe also don't describe any of the women they performed these early embryo transfers on. They don't even count them. There must have been hundreds. In the doctors' book, I sense their forms in the dark, just beyond the pages. The children they never had would be my age now.

THE DAY I TRIED to begin IVF—only to be told, several hours later, that I couldn't continue—I sat in the waiting room, watching the other women around me. Some leafed through magazines; others looked at their phones. It was seven in the morning, and many were dressed for work. We did not meet each other's eyes. This was stoicism *en masse*; we were training each other to keep it together. I filled out form after form on the clipboard, sensing the certainty of another woman a few rows away, her pen moving rapidly through the differently colored pieces of paper: *here*, and *here*, and *here*. She was inscribing her name with such force that I picked up my pace. I wasn't sure if it was bravery or passivity or both. This was what it looked like to give consent. Every time a nurse—always a woman—walked through the door, we all looked up. She would call a name. One woman would rise, clutching her bag to her, and through the doors she would go. The waiting room was tastefully decorated, deliberately domestic, full of upholstered chairs and table lamps, with mild-mannered abstractions on the walls. I was being trained to seat, literally, the anxiety I might feel, taught to be patient, to defer my own sense of time. Waiting to be seen, the main ontological event would be through those doors. I remember thinking that some of us beginning that day could be pregnant within a few weeks. I could feel my future branching. In a month, all could be the same or all could be changed.

You usually begin IVF on the second day of your period, and so when I was called to the examination room and asked to undress, I was embarrassed about the blood leaking out onto the sheet below me. I wasn't ashamed that I menstruated, but I had been taught, my entire life, to keep this blood hidden. Just as with the first introductory appointment, everyone averted their eyes. My doctor called out more numbers. He withdrew the ultrasound. I saw a flash of the bloody plastic sheath this time as the doctor peeled it off. They left me alone to dress: they could look at my blood, but they couldn't watch me put my bra back on.

When the nurse rang me that afternoon, and told me that I couldn't begin injecting myself, that my hormones did not bode well, that the doctor would ring the next morning, I fell into the internet. For the past fifteen years, I've spent at least four hours a day looking at a computer screen, but I had always bounced across it like a skipping stone, gathering information, unaware of my own momentum. Now, the internet became a whirlpool, a vast gray eye looking back at me, pulling my interest away from anything else. I could not work. I could not write. I could not watch a movie or a television show. All I could do was read thousands of messages on fertility boards, clicking the hours away, googling increasingly sophisticated Boolean phrases. For the rest of the month, I must've read close to a novel's worth of messages each day. Their words piled up in me, and still I read. I don't know what else I could have done. My mother was too upset to offer solace. My father didn't think it was the end of the world. I had not told my friends about freezing my eggs. No one I knew would have understood the weight of the nurse's words, or how it felt to see all my medication piled on the shelf unused.

Talking to the doctor on the phone about my FSH results, I heard the doubt in his voice. They could test my numbers again in a month's time. Yes, the results could change. But a poor FSH and AMH reading are like storm clouds on the horizon; something is *off*. I heard the disconnection in his tone. I was no longer a viable patient. I would not help him maintain his clinic's excellent implantation rate.

Throughout the 1970s, Edwards and Steptoe encountered a number of problems. The negative publicity had generated more interest, including offers of financial support from foundations and private donors, and this had allowed them to set up a larger lab in Oldham, but their rate of fertilized embryos dipped for reasons they couldn't discern. The hormone regimen they were prescribing women did not seem to prepare the uterine lining well for implantation. And there were other distractions: Edwards was elected as city councilor for Cambridge, and he stopped commuting as much to Oldham. Steptoe's arthritis was becoming progressively worse, and the pain in his hip made it hard for him to work. He was due to retire in 1978. Purdy was nursing her mother through cancer. For nine months in the mid-1970s, they did not work at all, before starting to experiment, yet again, with differing percentages of progesterone, estrogen, and hCG. There were a number of heartbreakingly close calls. In 1975, they actually obtained a positive pregnancy result for one woman, despite her history of infections and surgery, but after seven weeks, it became clear that it was ectopic. (The embryo had implanted in the stump of her scarred fallopian tube, rather than in the uterus, and had to be removed.) Another pregnancy shortly afterward also ended in miscarriage. These patients' reactions aren't described in the book. Edwards and Steptoe focused on their progress step by step, their gaze barely beyond the next task. They discovered the problem with their culture; their supply of liquid paraffin, which they used to suppress evaporation, had become toxic. Their rate of fertilization and cleavage increased again. There was another miscarriage. They decided to remove all hormone dosages, and simply rely on the body's natural ovulation of one egg, no matter if it occurred in the middle of the night. Edwards theorized that if they tracked a surge of luteinizing hormone—which the brain produces, triggering ovulation—they might have some advance warning. They had no idea if success was within arms' reach, or hundreds of miles away.

I found another clinic, further uptown, who had a doctor in it who specialized in women with high FSH. The appointment was three weeks away. If he took me on, I would begin almost immediately, and so I did everything I could to lower my FSH. Acupuncture was supposed to help, so I made an appointment with a doctor in traditional Chinese medicine. It was summer, and I cycled through New York City, sweating. Her office was in midtown, in an anonymous building. Another waiting room, this time with a large bulletin board covered with baby announcement cards. They had subdivided a tiny space into eight minuscule consultation rooms. The doctor moved from one to another, aided by many smiling assistants. She listened to me, but was obviously watching for different things. She examined my tongue, felt my pulse with a hand as small as a child's. I had an imbalance of energy, she said. I would need to stop the hot yoga. I would need to slow down. She would prescribe tea for me to drink morning and night. She asked me to undress and lie down. I was growing used to the sound of paper rustling beneath me.

Before she began her acupuncture, they cupped me, which involved lighting alcohol swabs inside small glass cups, then quickly attaching them one by one to my lower back. The suction formed by the vacuum of oxygen draws blood to that area of the body. I lay on my stomach, and they set a timer for ten minutes, turned off the lights and withdrew. If I moved at all, the glass cups would shift and tinkle against each other. I felt like a fragile stegosaurus. I could hear the sounds of other women's voices in the other rooms. They sounded happy. My eyes were leaking, a slow ooze of sadness.

The cups came off with a delicious sucking noise. The doctor came. With firm, quick movements, she inserted needles into my head, earlobes, stomach, hands and legs. Tap Tap. Tap Tap. "Meditate on your womb," she said, then turned the lights off again, this time for thirty minutes.

I had the strong sense of entering a fairy tale. My body was a vast palace, but here was a room in which time seemed to have sped up. The furniture in there was light with age. A witch is not a woman with special powers. A witch is a woman who has lost her powers, who has to resort to spells and potions. ·

I cycled home, and drank her bitter tea.

I considered, frantically, other options. Adoption. Embryo adoption. Years later, when I read about Edwards and Steptoe's development of IVF, I recognized, with a bitter pang, their comment that they encountered a surfeit of women willing to go under the knife in 1971 when they began their first embryo transfers with patients. These women knew the odds of falling pregnant were extraordinarily low, and yet they persisted in volunteering. In my state, I was willing to do anything as long as it meant that I was moving, deciding, fighting. Any decision felt better than none. I couldn't adopt in the United States if I wasn't a citizen, and so I began the process to convert my green card into citizenship. I had always been wary to do so: now I didn't hesitate.

Twice a week that month, I cycled into midtown, undressed in one of the consultation rooms, lay down, and waited for the doctor to come see me. She would ask me to stick out my tongue, feel my pulse again. "Aah," she would politely say, and make a note in my chart.

"Better?" I'd ask.

"Yes," she'd say.

Sometimes I fell asleep with the needles in. When they came to remove them, the assistants would often stroke my hair, giving me a tiny caress that always started up my tears again.

I continued to obsessively read online, and learned the dialect of my condition. Acronyms proliferated to such a degree that glossaries had sprung up. Some of this had to do with a kind of coyness about apparently gross events. A period was AF (Aunt Flo). Sex was a BD (Baby Dance) or a DTD (Do the Deed). Women endlessly debated numbers with each other: How many IVF rounds did you go through? How much weight did you put on? What was your FSH number? At times, it felt close to a pure number sequence: 8, 4, 2, 0. How many eggs were removed, how many fertilized, how many implanted? Did you give birth? Emoticons proliferated. What would've looked nearly incomprehensible to me even a month before now made sense:

> Me 40 (just turned) DH 42 TTC 2 yrs
> Oct 2011-IUI #1: 1 folli—canceled:-(
> Nov 2011-IUI #2: 2 folli, HCG trigger, prog tablets = BFN
> Feb 2012-IUI #3: natural cycle, HCG trigger, insemination
> mistimed (thanks a lot)—BFN
> Apr 2012-IVF #1: Getting ready for IVF with donor egg—
> DE from sister who is 38 yrs, yikes! (it was all we were
> comfortable with, she is older but everything looks good—
> fingers crossed) May 29: 2 Embies . . . 2WW! BFN—wasn't
> meant to be

This was a forty-year-old woman, married to a forty-two-year-old man. They had been trying to conceive for two years. She had undergone three intrauterine inseminations (IUIs), likely stimulated by hormones. The first was canceled because only one follicle developed, and presumably the cost couldn't be justified. For the second insemination she had two follicles, and was given an hCG trigger shot (a massive dose of human chorionic gonadotropin that stimulates ovulation at a precise time). She took progesterone tablets to develop her uterine lining so that an embryo could successfully implant, but nothing did. The third IUI went the same way, but they mistimed the insemination (there's a reasonably tight time frame between the administration of the hCG shot and when an egg is

released from the ovaries). She then tried IVF with her sister's donated eggs. They succeeded in creating two embryos, which were
transferred into her uterus on May 29. She waited two weeks, and
got a BFN (a Big Fat Nothing), rather than a BFP (a Big Fat Positive).

The women in the waiting room of my clinic never seemed to
speak to one another, but online, everyone reached out across time
and space. In many ways, it was remarkable. This was a way of dealing with the asymmetry between clinical science and patient experience: if they could not be visible to their doctor, they could be to
each other. These were their expedition notes, their encounters with
science. All of those unnamed women that Edwards and Steptoe experimented on (or with)—the *throng*—were lost to the public record, but these women weren't. You could read a conversation that
was five or six years old. The events described *must* have passed, but
here were multiple transmissions, still moving through deep space
on the internet, permanently capturing motion and uncertainty.

I didn't post. I didn't feel like I belonged. I didn't trust the coyness: it felt prudish, insistently heterosexual. I didn't trust the baby
talk. "May your embie be sticky." "Baby dust for everyone." There
was a fairly strict emotional script that appeared to be a given. Grief,
joy, and that was it. I didn't trust the swift and rapid tonal shifts. At
the end of many of their messages, these women would append an
electronic signature, often peppered with visual icons that summed
up their progress to date: a stork carrying a baby, along with birth
dates in blue for a boy, or pink for a girl. The posters' zest for microdistinctions seemed a calling card of enthusiasts, rather than critics,
and I realized that even in this moment, I could not stop being the
latter. Overwhelmingly, these women were white, American, and
married. They could afford the treatment, which still cost thousands

of dollars with good health insurance. These women belonged to a very particular economic and racial niche, which seemed to pass without remark. The boards did not question the basic assumptions behind IVF. They did not consider the root of one's baby lust. What about all the women who couldn't afford this? What about all the people who knew not to bother, that pregnancy just wasn't going to be an option?

As I read, and drank tea, and cycled, and had needles inserted into my body, and grieved, all over and over again, I also made a series of choices that felt hypothetical at the time, but were far from it. I had thought to freeze my eggs, but now, it seemed very unlikely I could harvest enough to freeze, then successfully thaw, fertilize, and implant. The surer bet was to create an embryo, and implant that, right away, no freezing required. That, of course, required sperm. I looked up sperm donation banks, but upon reflection, decided that if I *could* give the kid a biological father who'd be present, I preferred that option, in spite of all its emotional complexities. I knew two men willing to donate sperm, to essentially co-parent, and I talked it over with both of them. For one man, it was clear that he wouldn't mind our relationship beginning again. I think he thought donating sperm was an unusual but highly effective way to reconnect. For the other man, there was no question of any kind of sexual relationship: we were each done with that. Shahzad and I had dated for seven years, and had been broken up for three. I knew him at his worst, and knew I could deal with it. I also knew he badly wanted to be a father. I decided it was far better to go with the relationship that felt the most stable, the one without any romance involved.

My decision was both highly pragmatic and impulsive. There are many people who would disagree with my logic, and for good reason. But given the circumstances, it was the best choice I could've made for myself. My rationale was so different from the women on the boards, who all seemed to be married, who described how they had always wanted to be mothers, ever since they were children themselves. If I'd had the presence of mind, I would've looked up queer fertility message boards and seen how other people were creating other kinds of kinship relationships, but I didn't. I just waited for my next period to arrive.

When I met my new doctor, it was with Shahzad, and together, we sat across the table from him. We lied and said we had been trying to conceive for six months. I gave them a list of the medications I already had on my shelves at home. We had genetic testing done. We talked through the results. The nurses frequently referred to Shahzad as my husband. The first few times I corrected them but after a while, I gave up. We benefited from the misperception; in New York State, there are more testing hurdles for donor sperm than a partner's sperm, and we felt we had no time to lose. In a month where time appeared to stand still, when it felt like all I did was wait, we changed both of our lives irrevocably.

The tone of Steptoe and Edwards's memoir significantly changes when they describe their first meeting with Lesley and John Brown—indeed, Lesley is the first patient out of thousands, by this time, that they actually name. The Browns had been referred to Steptoe by their gynecologist. They had been trying to have a child for ten years, but Lesley had blocked fallopian tubes. Steptoe's assessment of her at their first appointment was approving: he wrote, "She was quietly determined, strong in resolve, unlikely to panic, and would suffer whatever was necessary with stoicism." It is his first and only character portrait of a patient in his book.

Louise Brown, in her own memoir *My Life as the World's First Test-Tube Baby*, offers more context. Her parents were far from the stereotypical model of white privilege. Both John and Lesley left school at fourteen and began a string of menial jobs. Both came from broken homes. On the night they first met each other at the pub (when Lesley was sixteen), they ended up sleeping rough in a railway carriage. Their early days together were spent on welfare and drinking down at the local pub. Eventually, John obtained a job as a bus conductor and they moved into a house, inching their way up into the working class, buying a house in Bristol. When they were referred to Steptoe, it was through the National Health Service. Though he explained the procedure, Lesley later said that she was entirely unaware that the new technique she was about to try had never been successful before.

A few days after we saw the second doctor, my period came. I went in to give blood and undergo another ultrasound. That afternoon, there was a message on my phone. Another nurse. "Your FSH is 9. You are going to start treatment tonight." And just like that, I could begin. It happened to be exactly the thirty-seventh birthday of Louise Brown.

Those who've gone through this experience might be amazed by this change in my FSH. The doctors did not know why mine improved, or why it fluctuates in general. I rested, did acupuncture, drank that herbal tea. It felt like a miracle—and I did not stop, simply turned to the next step, and began to open the boxes of medicine on my shelf.

IN 1905, THE physiologist Ernest Starling delivered a lecture in London in which he proposed the word *hormone* (derived from the Greek word meaning "to arouse or excite") to describe his theory about "chemical messengers" that sped from "cell to cell along the bloodstream," and which "may coordinate the activities and growth of different parts of the body." His willingness to name and clarify biological action at a distance begat what's since been called "the golden age of endocrinology." Scientists rushed to identify the chemical structures of different hormones, noting where they were produced in the body, and what their effect was. In the 1920s, the American scientist Edgar Allen set out to identify the particular hormones produced by the ovary. He was one of the first scientists to understand that the egg matured and grew as a result of a mammal's fluctuating hormones. Estrogen and progesterone were isolated and characterized. Understanding the endocrinology of a biological woman might be the first step to understanding how to either improve ovulation, or stop it. In the late 1940s, Piero Donini, an Italian scientist, was able to extract and purify FSH and LSH, the hormones that stimulate ovulation. He also discovered that the highest levels of these hormones were actually in post-menopausal women, and theorized that as women aged, and their egg production declined, the body attempted to help stimulate ovulation with more and more FSH and LSH. If you were to treat women suffering from infertility with the two hormones in combination—with a drug he termed "Pergonal"—they might be induced to ovulate more regularly.

Donini had no way of producing or marketing Pergonal, and so his paper announcing the discovery languished for a decade until the Viennese-born, Israeli-educated researcher Bruno Lunenfeld reached out to Donini. Lunenfeld, not yet graduated from medical school, and by his own account dedicated to increasing the Jewish population after the Holocaust, saw the potential of the drug, and began to contact pharmaceutical companies in an attempt to mount a clinical trial. One obvious hurdle was the fact they needed daily urine from at least 400 menopausal women. One of the companies most interested was the Italian pharmaceutical company Serono, which happened to include the nephew of Pope Pius XII on the executive board. The Vatican also owned 25 percent of Serono. Pope Pius XII personally intervened, requesting that nunneries across Italy supply their urine to Serono, which hauled it in tanker trucks to Rome. It took ten nuns ten days to produce enough urine for one treatment: 600 nuns were conscripted for the trial. In 1962, a woman treated by Lunenfeld with Pergonal in Tel Aviv gave birth to a baby girl; within two years there were another twenty pregnancies. By the mid-1980s, demand outstripped the nuns' supply, and Serono began to synthesize the hormones in the lab.

The drugs I injected myself with that first evening, Follistim and Menopur, were gonadotropins, descendants of Pergonal. Both drugs stimulated the ovaries into maturing multiple follicles at once. In a normal, un-stimulated cycle, only one follicle—maybe two—would mature. This time, all of them would grow, and then, in two weeks, all would be aspirated from my body. I was taking high doses because of my FSH. Follistim came in an injection pen, the dose delivered into my stomach fat. The website stated it was "man-made," which seemed an indirect way of saying they probably used recombinant DNA, though it was unclear whether the DNA was produced via animal, virus, or bacteria. The drug companies' aversion to outlining their processes is not surprising: beyond intellectual property issues, patients may be squeamish about the origins of the drugs they're injecting into themselves. Menopur was prepared by dissolving a vial of powder into a vial of diluent, which was then injected, using a longer needle, into my thigh. Menopur is still made from the urine of postmenopausal women; ironically, the information leaflet *assured* me of this fact. I wondered about the women on the other end of this vast global supply chain, peeing into containers, as I watched the powder dissolve. Here I was, paying for hormone extract from women done with babies so that I could have one. It was harder to inject myself than I anticipated. In order to overcome my evolutionary instinct not to insert a sharp pointed metal object into myself, I had to talk out loud, to literally tell myself to push the plunger down. Each injection cost hundreds of dollars.

Two days later, I was back to the clinic, for more blood work and an ultrasound. Again, the following day. Again, two days later. As it took an hour to commute each way to the clinic, stimulating my ovaries became a part-time job. I grew used to blood being drawn, to lying on the examination chair and opening my legs. I started to sense a pattern in the numbers they called out, focusing the crosshairs on each follicle, larger than Leeuwenhoek's wildest dreams, moving, twitching, still alive. My body responded quickly—almost too quickly. Within a few days, one of my follicles was getting so big that the doctor told me to inject another drug to slow it down, to allow the others to catch up. I felt like Alice in Wonderland, eating her cake to grow, drinking from a little bottle to shrink. As my ovaries swelled, I felt increasingly full, like I had just eaten a large meal. I walked incessantly, miles and miles a day. Compared to other stories on the internet, I had it easy.

Lesley was not given hormones; Edwards and Steptoe had grown wary of using gonadotropins, and simply tracked her movement toward ovulation by measuring the estrogen and progesterone in her urine. She gathered it morning and night. Every day, they charted

what her body was already doing, waiting, hoping, trying to anticipate the best moment to operate and retrieve her egg.

Normally it takes ten to fourteen days for the follicles to grow to
size, but they scheduled me for surgery on the eighth day. They told
me the exact time to inject my hCG trigger shot, which would cause
me to ovulate in thirty-six hours. It was intramuscular—one of
those very large, long needles—and it needed to be injected into the
top fleshy part of the ass. I was to inject it at night, at eleven p.m.
There would be no more hCG if I messed it up. A friend came around,
and she practiced for a while on a banana with another needle,
learning to anticipate the resistance and give of flesh. Shahzad sat on
one side of the bed, watching us. I assured her that she could go slow,
take her time, that no matter how much it hurt, I wouldn't move.
And I didn't. The liquid dissipated, the ache in my ass declined.

On the day of retrieval, I sat in a waiting room at a hospital with
six other women, all dressed in hospital gowns, hair coverings, and
surgery socks. We silently waited to be harvested. I was the only one
without a man beside me. I took photographs on my phone of the
magazine covers in the waiting room. I wanted to show a future kid
the banality of the news on the day it was fertilized. Someone called
Bubba was on the cover of *Golf Digest*. Kaitlyn Jenner was called
Bruce Jenner, and had begun hormone therapy. I tried to do the
math. Six retrievals in one morning. The clinic worked seven days a
week and closed for four weeks a year (two weeks at a time). This
meant that this one clinic alone did more than 2,000 follicular aspi-
rations a year. The nurses and receptionists worked smoothly in
tandem, calling names, gathering belongings.

It was my first time *walking* as a patient into an operating room. I
was asked to climb up onto the table and lie back.

"The IV might burn a little," the anesthesiologist said. "It's going in now."

"Put your left leg up onto the stirrup," the nurse said, wrapping Velcro straps around it. I don't even remember lifting my right leg.

While I was unconscious, the surgeon inserted a catheter-like tube through my vagina, made a small incision into each of my ovaries, and sucked the follicular fluid out. When I read about the operation beforehand, I couldn't shake the description I'd once read in a cheap horror novel of a shark's stomach contents: a license plate, a bit of a boot, fish, and a man's torso. They also were removing my flotsam and jetsam. In reality, it does not look like that. You can now see a dissection of an ovary on YouTube. The flesh is the size of a flattened plum. A needle is inserted at several points, aspirating the contents of each follicle. The hand that does this work is quick, matter-of-fact, as knowing as a practiced cook chopping an onion.

When I woke up from my retrieval, it was to the other ex, smiling down at me. Shahzad had gone on tour, and because no one else in my life in New York City knew what I had decided to do, this ex was there to take me home. We went to lunch at a diner nearby; he had starved in solidarity, and we ordered tuna melts and watched the line cooks work in silence. I thought of my eggs five blocks away, disembodied, and Shahzad's sperm, swimming around each one. The human egg (the largest cell in the body) is forty times the size of a sperm (the tiniest cell); in images of conception, the egg appears as big as a child's ball, the sperm as small as sesame seeds crowding around it, tails whipping from side to side. Some of Shahzad's sperm might be still, obviously dead. Others might be gamely making an attempt, but weakening. I knew that whereas most readings of this image of conception tend to emphasize the spermatozoa's energy, the egg was also exerting an inexorable gravitational pull. The surface of an egg has adhesive molecules that hold the sperm's head tightly against it, just as the surface of the sperm also releases digestive enzymes. Ideally, the more the sperm wriggles (its side-to-side movement is ten times more powerful than its forward movement), the more the surface of the egg dissolves, guiding the sperm in the right direction.

This science, for all its numbers and percentages and studies, felt just as magical as the stories I read as a child. There is a story by Hans Christian Andersen called "Thumbelina," which begins: "There was once a woman who wished very much to have a little child, but she could not obtain her wish." I had never thought I would be that woman. In the story, she went to a fairy and asked for a child. "Oh, that can be easily managed," the fairy said, and gave her a magic barleycorn. The fairy's matter-of-fact tone reminded me of my doctor's. This could all be easily managed, even when it was obvious it couldn't.

That night, I lay awake and imagined my egg (was it an embryo now?) six miles away. There was magic in those incubators. Galaxies of human life were expanding and contracting, and among them were my—our—planets. It felt like a miracle, like a story about a man whose foot was chopped off, and the foot continued to hop about, and then away. My body had life beyond me.

I wasn't told until the next day what had really happened. Shahzad's sperm had pretty terrible mobility and morphology (the shape of the head), and the embryologist made the decision to use ICSI (intracytoplasmic sperm injection), a technique developed in the late 1980s. They selected a few sperm that did seem well-shaped and moving well, cut their tails off, and injected each one, using a micropipette, directly into my eggs. There are many videos on this process online. The egg looks like a balloon with a clearly visible "shell." When it is close to maturity, it divides its DNA into two sets of chromosomes, and the unneeded set—called the polar body—appears as a tiny bubble at the edge of the cell. Insertion needs to happen away from the polar body, and also away from the meiotic spindle (that pulls the chromosomes apart), which is not visible, but which is usually below the polar body. Using a micromanipulator, the embryologist holds the egg still with one pipette that applies gentle suction through a microinjector. With the other hand, she approaches the egg from the other side with a long thin pipette. Inside, you can see a single sperm slide toward its tip, immobilized. The pipette begins to steadily press against the outside wall of the egg, causing it to bulge sideways into an oval. Technicians are encouraged to not push hard and allow the needle to do its work with a minimum of pressure. Watching it, you can't help but hold your breath. Suddenly, the egg gives, and the needle enters, pauses, pulls backward now, to break a barely visible second inner membrane which is so elastic it can sometimes take ten or twenty seconds for the cell wall to give. When it does, the pipette pushes further in again, and the sperm is slowly expelled, along with the bare minimum of PVP, the viscous substance in which the sperm have been suspended for selection. The pipette withdraws, and taps the outside of the egg gently, almost lovingly.

They rang me the next day with the results. They had retrieved seven eggs. Six were mature. They were able to successfully fertilize five. I had my own number sequence. I called Shahzad. "I'm just so proud," he said, a little tearful, "that our bodies could do this." Science made those embryos, but the material came from us. We just about burst with happiness.

On the fifth day, I visited the hospital again, this time in the afternoon, for implantation. Once again, there were six women in the waiting room, all dressed in scrubs. There were the same magazines. But this time, the operating room had opera playing, and one whole wall had disappeared, to reveal an embryology lab behind it. I could see lab clinicians walking from incubator to lab bench and microscope carrying petri dishes, one hand beneath, the other resting protectively on top. I lay back and opened my legs yet again. I no longer cared how many people were in the room when this happened, or how bright the lights were. On the computer screen next to me, there was a magnified image of the two embryos they were going to put inside of me. They were blastocysts, exactly what Purdy had seen for the first time in 1970: cellular rubble at the edges, smoothness in the middle. "They're good-looking," the embryologist said, and I felt fierce pride. They gave me a photograph to take home and put on my mantelpiece. Edwards was right: they were beautiful. I had two weeks to wait.

IN THE 1980S, precisely as the IVF industry was rapidly expanding, a number of feminist critiques of new reproductive technologies were mounted by academics and writers, including Maria Mies, Janice Raymond, Renate Klein, Jalna Hanmer, and Robyn Rowland, who also formed FINRRAGE, the Feminist International Network of Resistance to Reproductive and Genetic Engineering. This first wave of feminist scholarship about IVF (which Charis Thompson

dates as occurring between 1984 and 1991) consistently emphasized IVF's structural stratification, and was quick to note how new
reproductive technologies confirmed a conservative, heterosexual,
consumer-oriented vision of a nuclear family rather than extending
or widening our understanding of kinship. FINRRAGE also pointed
out that throughout history, Black, brown, and poor bodies had
consistently been legislated against, experimented upon, dehuman-
ized, and disrespected, and noted that IVF didn't seem set to disrupt
this state of affairs at all. Those who had money had the right and
ability to challenge their infertility, and those who didn't, couldn't.
Wealth literally bred—and to hell with a country's obligations to all
of its citizens. Any experimentation was only in the service of perpetuating a status quo.

One of my favorite writers from this early period of FINRRAGE
is the journalist Gena Corea, who published *The Mother Machine* in
1985. In this book, Corea wrote about many of the same figures who
have appeared here—about Karl Ernst von Baer, Robert Edwards,
and Patrick Steptoe, even Antonij Leeuwenhoek. She was taking
aim at the medical and scientific industry, which she saw as innately
and unrepentantly patriarchal, and she was beautifully adamant.
She made *everything* connect. IVF was the latest in a long line of in-
sults that had upended matriarchal systems of power. For her, this
upending began when we developed from hunter-gatherer to agrar-
ian societies: "We established a vertical master/slave relationship
with animals. We took animals in. We fed them. We befriended
them. We killed them. We ate them. In the course of this betrayal,
the slaughter of beings we had first befriended, we killed some
sensitivity in ourselves." For her, human history was one long empathy leak. Corea saw the development of the animal husbandry

industry as directly prefiguring the development of the IVF industry, noting the technological transfer of knowledge (particularly
with embryo freezing and surrogacy), and pointed out how efficien-
cies of scale and expectations of profit would inevitably dehuman-
ize the experience of women. The cow, she wrote, is "one of the
oldest forms in which the ancient Goddess was known," but their
treatment by male farmers—who often used misogynistic rhetoric
to refer to recalcitrant cows as women, and who bragged about
"making babies"—was a sign of how men would use new reproductive technologies to "other," demean, and reduce women.

Corea's skepticism of the medical industry led her to important
conclusions. She emphasized the issue of consent, noting how few
studies carried out during this period even mentioned what consent
protocols were put in place. She called out Edwards and Steptoe,
among others. She named transgression. The first artificial insemination by donor (AID) in the historical record (carried out in 1884
by Dr. William Pancoast at Sansom Street Hospital in Philadelphia)
was performed on an unconscious woman who did not know she
had been inseminated by sperm from a medical student rather than
her husband. Corea identified this as a rape. She described John
Rock and Arthur T. Hertig's hysterectomies of women around 1940
at the Free Hospital for Women in Brookline, Massachusetts. The
women were not told that Rock and Hertig were also looking, during surgery, for implanted embryos (even *scheduling* the surgeries to
follow women's ovulation cycles without explaining why), and that
the removal of an embryo was, essentially, also performing an abortion without consent. (It should be noted that Rock and Hertig later
acknowledged that they were partially inspired in their reproductive research by Huxley's *Brave New World*.) Corea asked what con-

sent actually meant "in a society in which men as a social group control not just the choices open to women, but also women's motivation to choose." If those women in Brookline had been told of Rock and Hertig's plans, but if they had no other way to pay for this medical care, how freely given could their consent have been? Corea was quick to point out the financial implications of new reproductive technologies for any woman who was either poor or of color: society did not value her eggs, she wrote, but there "may well be a demand for her womb" as a surrogate. The tone of much of Corea's scholarship was remarkably, free-wheelingly, bravely unambiguous. To participate in any part of these new reproductive technologies was to cede your feminist convictions. Women like me were dupes. We had internalized a self-hating rhetoric. Our choice was not actually a choice at all. Our desire to breed was not even our own anymore.

Corea would understand my account of FSH and AMH numbers as entirely within the "interests of the patriarchy, reducing women to Matter." In her book, she continued: "Just as the patriarchal state now finds it acceptable to market parts of a woman's body (breast, vagina, buttocks) for sexual purposes in prostitution and the larger sex industry, so it will soon find it reasonable to market other parts of a woman (womb, ovaries, egg) for reproductive purposes." It was not just the body itself, but representations of it: Corea thought *any* form of medical image-making an objectification, an encouragement for a woman to think of her body as not-herself, to transpose herself from thinking subject to acted-upon object. Following her line of thinking, Edwards's use of the word *beautiful* to describe blastocysts, his attentive descriptions of them, are annexation in the guise of aestheticism. To declare something beautiful was to detach it, to separate it, and put it on a pedestal (or petri dish). My transvaginal ultrasounds—one after the other—were a training in dissociative thinking, in understanding my body as a set of parts. (Even my instinctive metaphors—wandering feet, galaxies—followed this dissociative spatial logic.) The *coup de grace*, of course, was the photograph of my blastocysts, given to me to put on my mantelpiece, to treasure—treasure!—as a crowning patriarchal metonymy: here *they* were, which used to be me, which was outside me for a time, but now was *back* inside. These shifting self-identifications could also be false recognitions, which for Corea, was precisely the destabilizing point: I was learning to distrust my own body, its wholeness, to only think of it in parts.

Feminists in the 1980s seized on fetal imaging as a particularly resonant example because it appears to contain a compounding set of objectifications. The woman undresses, and just like the figure of the nude in Western art, is transformed from being a naked human to being a type, an object for diagnosis. The sexual organs are a point of focus, but care is taken not to sexualize them (just as with a "tasteful" nude statue). Some modesty is insisted upon via the pointed specialization of the gaze. The ultrasound shows us the fetus inside, and that image immediately shifts the woman's body from foreground to background. Her objectifications literally nest inside one another.

Feminist anthropologists and sociologists have, in the main, agreed with this line of interpretation. Barbara Katz Rothman was one of the first to elaborate the aesthetic rhetoric of these sonograms, observing how the "fetus in utero has become a metaphor for 'man' in space, floating free, attached only by the umbilical cord to the spaceship." Marilyn Strathern argued that the mother became a "mere" environment, an "enabling technology.... The mother seems visible only as an appendage to the foetus, in the same way as nutrients are simply regarded as resources." For Corea, this followed a long-established tradition of conferring symbolic power on the sight of a woman's body, all the while undermining her legal and economic agency in the world.

It is very hard to *not* see this sleight of hand in the story of Lesley Brown, even in the account written by Edwards and Steptoe. It's striking how little Lesley participated in the decisions that were made about her pregnancy. She was not informed she was pregnant. It was Steptoe and Edwards's habit (which continued well into the 1980s) to ring the husband and inform him of the pregnancy test result, rather than the person on whom they had operated. When it became clear that the world's first IVF pregnancy was continuing, and Lesley moved from her first to second trimester, it was also her husband (along with Steptoe) who negotiated with the *Daily Mail* for exclusive rights to the coverage of the birth. Lesley was not informed of this deal. When she was admitted to hospital close to her due date, reporters dressed as boiler repairmen, plumbers, window cleaners, and priests roamed the hospital grounds, trying to bribe staff. One journalist even rang in a bomb scare, halting several operations and requiring an evacuation of the hospital (including women actually in labor). Lesley wasn't given any newspapers for fear the printed speculation would unnerve her. The windows to her hospital room were covered. Everyone thought it in her best interests to keep her literally in the dark.

This paternalism was in part a reaction to the extraordinary nature of the events. Steptoe and Edwards kept Brown's impending cesarean operation a secret from almost everyone; on the day,

Lesley pretended to eat all of her lunch so that even her daytime nursing staff would be none the wiser. Her husband wasn't told until an hour before the operation, and her catheter was inserted by torchlight, so that reporters wouldn't identify her room. When she was wheeled to the operating theater close to midnight, police officers lined the corridors, in case the press stormed the hospital. Lesley was given a general anesthetic, and so it was Edwards and Steptoe, not Lesley, who first witnessed Louise's birth. In their book, Edwards described Steptoe's incisions step by step: the opening of the abdomen, the slitting of the sac. "A firm hoist and out came the head through the 'letter-box' opening. Baby's face was looking upwards and towards me," he wrote. Steptoe pushed down on Lesley's stomach, and the baby's shoulders appeared, like a pea being squeezed out of a pod. "Left hand under the buttocks and out she came," he added. It was 11:47 p. m. on July the 25th, 1978: "Glorious. She was chubby, full of muscular tone. The cord was pulsating strongly although it was hooked round the left thigh. I held the head low and we sucked and cleared the mouth and throat. She took a deep breath. Then she yelled and yelled and yelled." You can still hear the relief in Edwards and Steptoe's words, their exaltation at life. It is the first moment in their book you sense their own love as parents, their deep satisfaction at the joy they could create for another couple. You can also hear how they set Lesley aside. It is striking how unaware Edwards and Steptoe are of the ways in which they—with all the best intentions in the world—repeatedly undermined her agency.

Lesley found it difficult to resume her life as a new mother. Not surprisingly, she found the scrutiny jarring. She couldn't leave her house for weeks after the birth because of the media scrum outside.

She received thousands of cards, telegrams, and poems from around the world. Hundreds of women wrote to her about their own experience of infertility. One sent her a bloody test tube. One of Louise's earliest memories was of being passed over the back fence to a neighbor in order to avoid a photographer's lens.

Throughout the last four decades, hundreds of academics have been committed to exposing structural inequities in reproductive technologies, along with the ways in which women are deprived of agency in their reproductive choices. Their ethnographic studies are accurate and pressing, but this work doesn't come up in basic key term searches on the internet, and their findings are not reflected in clinical literature, how-to guides, or even in pamphlets at IVF clinics. Most women are unaware that this valley system of knowledge exists. If I were a betting woman, I would be happy to wager that none of the women sitting in those waiting rooms alongside me had ever heard of FINRRAGE or the hundreds of books that warn of the physical and ethical dangers of reproductive technologies. I have spent a lot of time wondering why. It seems quite possible to remain unmoved when your own subjugation is pointed out. IVF came about through centuries of men looking and seeing women's bodies as objects—there is no way around this fact, and it has shaped women's experiences of their own fertility—but when a woman is contemplating IVF, the concern (at least in patient-centered literature) is not whether this treatment enacts a centuries-long system of patriarchal objectification, but whether her odds are good. The history of our bodies that is easily available to us was not written by us, but that has not appeared to slow people down for even a second as they contemplate becoming a guinea pig or a moral pioneer or a spacewoman, depending on your point of view. Both

Lesley and I—and many others—are driven by grief and fear and desire to take a course of action that is hard enough to endure, let alone question at the same time.

This desire is *old*. Many fairy tales are set in motion by a *deus ex femina*, by a woman who decides to take an unorthodox, experimental course of action to gain a child. In that sense, infertility is an occasion for storytelling. But that choice is often then quickly set aside; the mother in Andersen's "Thumbelina" is merely the springboard to the narrative, the occasion for the tiny slim-waisted woman to be brought into existence. In the fifth paragraph, Thumbelina is abducted—by another mother (this time a toad) to marry her son. The engine of the story is a series of abductions or coercions, as Tiny deals with one animal suitor after another. This isn't, of course, how the tale is generally explained. Most people would want to linger on Tiny's kindness to a bird, and how he repays her by carrying her away to a man with whom she *wants* to fall in love. But it is hard to avoid the insistent implication that a woman's movement in the world is tied to her partnering. And for me, it is hard to let go of how quickly we are encouraged to forget the mother, back at the beginning, who had waited, and wished, and waited, and wished, and risked, only to lose everything.

The media attention did not dissipate with Louise Brown's birth. Having negotiated one deal with the *Daily Mail*, John Brown decided to try to manage it further, and set up a number of press tours around the world, including a trip to Japan. It is unclear again how much say Lesley Brown had in this. In her own memoir, Louise describes her mother's increasing discomfort. The Browns took the money, but the interviews didn't become easier; if anything, John and Lesley found themselves increasingly monosyllabic in front of the world's media. Lesley was not willing to repeat the story of Louise's conception and birth *ad nauseam*. Her mute resistance was not acknowledged or respected, but perceived as a failure. As Louise later put it, "Why should a lorry driver from Bristol and his wife, who had worked in an underwear factory, suddenly make interesting television just because they had a baby?" Working out how to look after a child was consuming enough; Lesley herself just wanted to move on. She was grateful; she had gotten what she wanted. Now was not the time to look back. Her own narrative is obscured, and she slowly vanished from public view. She had waited, and wished, and waited, and wished, and risked, only to gain everything, but at a price it may have felt uncharitable to articulate.

7

WOMB WITH A VIEW

My father worked for more than thirty years at the University of Auckland's School of Medicine, but he wasn't a doctor, and didn't attend medical school as a student. He had trained as a biologist, and wrote his dissertation on the circadian rhythms of freshwater crayfish. When my parents returned with me from England, he found that no one was hiring biologists. He applied for a tutoring job in human embryology at the University of Auckland, reasoning that the processes which operate during early human development are common to all vertebrates, and that maybe his lack of specialist knowledge would not be viewed as a disadvantage. It also happened that the dean of the medical school had just bought a boat, and had no one else to talk to about sailing. My father—who had spent much of the previous decade building a boat himself and sailing it round the world—was hired.

Despite backing his way into the profession, and considering himself an introvert with no ambition to gain tenure or rise through the departmental ranks, my father became a dedicated teacher, relentless in developing creative ways for students to memorize and learn vast amounts of information. He created mnemonics and color-coding activities, played videos and recited poems, and constructed an echo chamber of esoteric references for his students, who learned about Romantic poetry, Civil War surgical miracles, and polar explorers in order to memorize the chambers and valves of the heart, or the digestive processes of the gut. His students loved him for focusing so deliberately on their own learning needs. In order to teach human embryo development, he designed a learning module in which students each made a four-week-old embryo out of modeling clay that showed, in different clay colors, the developing blood and nervous systems. He taught this unit for years: all over Auckland, there must've been thousands of these embryos, balanced on bookshelves and dressers. As a teenager, I stood by his own bookcase in his office, examining his personal copy.

It is no surprise that I think about my father when I read Gena Corea's description of a quasi-conspiracy among male scientists to subjugate women. It is easy to find men in history who had misogynistic views. Corea focused on Nobel Prize winners like Dr. Hermann J. Muller, a Marxist geneticist who in 1935 anticipated the possibility of frozen-sperm banks, and suggested that women only inseminate themselves with sperm of "transcendently estimable" men. Muller suggested that this sperm would have to be embargoed for decades after a man's death to assess a) how his children turned out, and b) if his achievements were all that estimable. If they were, and if women only gave birth to children from this sperm, in a century or two Muller thought the population could have "the innate quality of such men as Lenin, Newton, Leonardo, Pasteur, Beethoven, Omar Khayyám, Pushkin, Sun Yat-Sen, Marx. . . ." It would appear the future would be all-male, and mostly white. This idea was actually realized in 1976, when a California businessman established a sperm bank (in Muller's name) containing only Nobel Prize–winning sperm, and including samples from Dr. William Shockley, who had won the Nobel Prize for developing the transistor radio, and who turned out to be very unambiguously racist. Shockley's views were shocking, but he was part of a surprisingly extensive tradition of Nobel Prize winners offering both retrograde and radical takes on societal restructuring. (For example, the discoverer of DNA, Francis Crick, didn't see why people should have the right to have children. He wondered if the government could put something in food that would render the population automatically sterile, unless they paid a kind of breeding tax. At the very least, he thought, there should be a licensing scheme.) Corea, of course, had a field day with all of this. She concluded her chapter with the portentous words, "These are top scientists speaking. Men with power." The implication was clear.

Corea's synthesizing energy is deeply appealing to me because her desire to make everything connect amounts to a paradigm shift, but it is also, of course, difficult to reconcile her fear with my father. He is soft-spoken, contemptuous of bureaucracy, interested in humanizing the body rather than dehumanizing it. My father did not raise me to be a wife or a mother, or even to be particularly compliant. He raised me on books by explorers, on cycling and hiking. If he had any machismo, it was an asceticism I inherited: a certain hardness, a certain coldness. It could be identified as male, but it doesn't have to be. When he experienced a recurring ventricular tachycardia a few years ago, doctors from across the hospital system in Auckland kept turning up at his bed in his ward: everyone wanted to say hello. Many of the surgeons, residents, specialists, and doctors there had at one point taken his class. They recited his analogies back to him. They still had their embryo. My father has taught dissecting labs, where women's bodies were used, but it's *how* he taught which seems not to be accounted for in Corea's condemnation.

After my egg removal, I was instructed to begin my progesterone shots, which would aid any embryo implantation by developing the uterine lining. These shots were intramuscular, like the hCG, again with wickedly long needles, again in the upper fleshy part of my ass. Previously, that had felt a difficult enough maneuver to ask my friend to do it. Now I had no choice but to learn. I would have to inject myself every night for two weeks and then, if I was pregnant, for four weeks after that.

Each night, I stood with my back to my floor-length mirror, needle in hand. The first few days, I had to mark the spot on my skin with a pen; it helped me focus as I craned my head and arm around. The progesterone was kept in oil, which meant it was thicker to inject (and more painful). The Follistim pen that I'd begun with now felt like a joke, a tiny nip. I thought of Thumbelina's mother, and the fairy. "Oh, that can be easily managed," it told her. I was managing it. My syringes and pads and wipes were stacked neatly on my bookshelf, next to the medical waste disposal bin. My enchanted barleycorns.

One night, I must've hit an artery with the needle, and when I removed it, a thin arc of blood jetted out, spraying the mirror. It took a second for me to realize it would not stop on its own. More blood. I numbly stopped it with a finger and waited, wondering how long it would take for my body to repair itself. Only a few minutes, it turned out.

In her book *The Politics of Reproduction* (1981), much cited at the

time, the philosopher Mary O'Brien argued that medical procedures during pregnancy were an attempt by men to disrupt a woman's reproductive consciousness. Men, she said, had a discontinuous
experience of reproduction: he ejaculates, and nine months later a
child is born. There is no certainty it is his, and to connect the two
acts is "an intellectual act": paternity is an "abstract idea." Women,
on the other hand, had a continuous experience: they participate in
intercourse, grow the embryo and fetus during nine months of
pregnancy, birth a child, then feed it milk from their bodies. There is
no point where the woman is separated from the reality of reproduction. O'Brien and others suggested that the male desire to disrupt this reality was an attempt to undermine female power, to
co-opt and control what was not theirs. A patriarchal world of new
reproductive technologies was man-made—a promising, if seemingly unintentional pun. FINRRAGE's "Declaration of Comilla,"
issued in 1989, aligned men with machines, engineering, and a
deductive thought pattern: the assumption that a thing "can be broken down into its components, analysed and put back." By contrast,
women were natural, not easily measured or quantified, seen as
subjective. Women were "compassionate, humane, and ecologically
sustainable." Following this line of reasoning, new reproductive
technologies created *more* discontinuity for women, because they
constantly drew attention to the ways in which a woman did not
know what was going on inside her body. A woman's way of knowing was ceded to male interpretive systems, to waiting for blood
work and scans to verify a reality.

On infertility message boards, the 2WW—two-week wait—is
the period of time between ovulation and your next period, which

is the time you wait in order to find out if you're pregnant: if sex, or an IUI (insemination by catheter), or an embryo transfer (the result of IVF) has actually worked. The uncertainty and the waiting are universally understood as a torture. The 2WW is part of a broader reorganization of time, a development of the art of waiting. I had spent that summer waiting: waiting to start, then waiting for my next period, then waiting for retrieval, then waiting for transfer, and now waiting for implantation. It could be that nothing had actually changed. It could be that everything had. Those first few days after transfer, the knowledge that two living creatures were inside me was strong; it colored everything like a kind of light filter. As the days passed, it became a binary: the embryos were dead or alive, and even if they were alive, they might be chromosomally abnormal; statistically speaking, 50 percent of a thirty-five-year-old woman's eggs are abnormal.

Online, there are many articles about how to bear the seemingly endless stretch of days (television, treating yourself, new cooking techniques, tackling small jobs), but they all seemed to miss what makes the two-week wait particularly unbearable, which is the fact that women suffering fertility issues go through this experience over and over again. In a two-week wait, it is tempting to avoid social occasions where people will ask how you are. You cannot drink. You are unusually risk-averse. As if you were ill, you are strangely deliberate about what to do with your energy. Do you dare jump into that waterhole? What about staying in the sun all day, dehydrated and hungry? The hope that you are pregnant slowly begins to build, like algal bloom in a pond. You inspect your breasts. Are they bigger? Every stomach twinge is interpreted as implantation cramps. You never thought of yourself as a nauseated person, but now you feel butterflies all of the time. It's hard to organize holidays or plane flights. You are constantly delaying decisions. You try to avoid calculating your due date, and fail. And then at the end of two weeks, you might find out that you weren't really waiting; you are not pregnant, and you were not really living your life the way you wanted to, and now those two weeks are gone and it's time to start all over again. You are always postponing your life for another that may never come. This feels like a profoundly discontinuous way of living. It requires a reassessment of how you understand momentum in your life, of how much the future provides some kind of scaffolding for the present.

I had practiced yoga for many years, and thought I knew my body fairly well. I had grown proficient at isolating my awareness to particular parts; I understood, for example, when I stood a certain way, how the ribs on my right side were working in relation to the inward rotation of my left thigh. But this did not help me now. I did not know what was going on inside of me. My body was not speaking to me yet. I felt utterly normal, and was terrified of what that meant. Before IVF, time sluiced through me like a waterfall. Now, I felt more like an old-fashioned water mill. The minutes filled me up, like drops of water in a cup at the end of each paddle. Time moved so slowly, adding, and adding, and adding—till I brimmed, then over I went again, with a splash.

These feelings are all very real for people who aren't undergoing IVF, who are simply trying to fall pregnant, as well; which is why O'Brien's distinction between a (male) discontinuity and (female) continuity of experience appears, on closer inspection, to overlook a set of meaningful complications. There is little room in her argument for nonbinary or trans people. Yes, one's anxiety is certainly heightened by the cost of IVF: a natural pregnancy is prefaced by sex or low-fi insemination with a turkey baster, and an IVF pregnancy is prefaced by appointments, scans, injections, surgery, etc. But the two-week wait only makes more visible the fact that in the first four months, a woman cannot feel the fetus's movements. She may discern she is pregnant from other symptoms—morning sickness, fatigue, a sensitivity to smell, tender breasts—but all of these can be attributed to hormonal changes rather than to the fetus. The cellular big bang going on inside her is largely undetectable. At that stage, even if she is pregnant, it can also feel like an abstract, even discontinuous idea.

Indeed, this uncertainty could be said to be a fundamental part of living, regardless of gender or pregnancy. There is a remarkable cognitive dissonance between our conception of bodily knowledge—the signals our body has of fatigue, hunger, or desire—and the world of cellular formation and degeneration. We do not know ourselves at a biological level; it is even hard to visualize the blood and flesh below the skin, the way our organs fold into each other, the composition of fat, blood, vein, and muscle. Our love of on-screen physical violence, particularly decapitations, amputations, arterial spray, or disembowelment, is a consequence-free way to remind ourselves of the existence of our insides. Our corporeality is remarkably easy to forget—so easy, in fact, that one senses an evolutionary advantage of some kind to putting aside the knowledge that your heart has beaten fifty times reading this paragraph. Our experience in our bodies is often discontinuous, and that doesn't have to be a patriarchal thing.

At the end of my two-week wait, I was on holiday in Maine. I was expecting the nurse's call, and knew I was going to be somewhere mundane, but I was still surprised when the phone rang and I found myself standing in an outdoor gear store, in between the Therm-a-Rests and camping stoves. I was embarrassed to answer the phone so politely, to wait for her to say something. I wanted to scream. Tell me! Tell me!

I was pregnant. But the nurse was cautious. My hCG—the hormone that over-the-counter pregnancy tests measure—was "lower," she said, "than I would like." I would need to take another blood test at the local hospital in two days, and the amount of hCG would need to at least double in that time.

I was ecstatic, literally hopping up and down with happiness. I tried to continue the holiday: hiked, ate lobster, fought off low fog and mosquitoes. In two days, I returned to Bar Harbor, and killed time between the blood draw and the results with shopping, watching families on holiday, daring to directly look, for the first time in months, at babies.

The nurse called again in the afternoon. I knew straight away from her tone. My hCG had risen, but not enough. It turned out you could be sort-of pregnant. It was likely that the embryo had implanted, but that it had chromosomal abnormalities. She told me I would miscarry, probably within the next two weeks. I returned to New York that day, holiday forgotten. All I could think about was the blood to come.

For the second phase of feminist scholarship about reproductive technologies—from 1992 to 2001—academics had been studying working IVF clinics for more than a decade, and so their data was about the lived experience of people. Earlier, more abstract claims about the industry grew more tempered. Doctors were discovered to be rather mixed in their motivations; it was acknowledged that they could have been patients at some point, too, might have also experienced how one's internal schema is altered when looking at one's body on a screen in twitching, pulsing real time. They might also know how it felt to give themselves up to a treatment process, how the future was put on hold until they found out if their body had done what they wanted it to do (healed, conceived, expelled, etc.). More critical attention was paid to kinship structures created by queer and nonbinary parents, and the number of clinics willing to work with single women and queer and gay couples increased.

In this second phase, too, more credit was given to patients in learning to navigate and manipulate their systems of treatment. In her book *Making Parents*, Charis Thompson argued that patients *actively* managed their objectification, engaging in it consciously for periods of time. Thompson reached this conclusion by interviewing a number of women, some who failed to fall pregnant and were still in treatment, and others who failed at first, then succeeded. She identified a number of patterns. When a woman was still in treatment, she was more likely to identify failure or success as reliant on a part of the process—faulty sperm, faulty egg, blocked tubes, etc.— thus objectifying that part of the body as something quite distinct. It was a mechanistic view of fertility. If that cycle did not result in a pregnancy, and there was no satisfying explanation for the failure, she could turn to think more broadly about the ethos of the clinic, or how she felt as a patient. If the women voluntarily objectified themselves in the first instance, they were now quick to sense the ways they were "just a number" in the second. But once they fell pregnant, their reasons for why they fell pregnant weren't strikingly mechanistic, and instead less causal, allowing for more subjectivity: "I just had a better feeling about it," one woman said. Women were more willing to remember how they felt in their own bodies, rather than how they appeared, more willing to not know, to acknowledge luck. These interpretations were by nature retroactive, which meant that Thompson's framing of objectification was intrinsically subjective. She was willing for the differences between these forms of objectification to be slight but crucial, writing, for instance, "The patients do not so much let themselves be treated like objects to comply with the physician as they comply with the physician to let themselves be treated like objects."

My miscarriage never happened. More blood tests revealed that the hCG was still rising: not enough to indicate any kind of viable pregnancy, but in such a way that my body did not know to expel the embryo. I waited one week, two weeks, three weeks, imagining this tiny collection of cells inside of me, still alive but lost, like a blindfolded person headed off in the wrong direction. I found myself measuring where I would've been had the pregnancy been healthy. By now there would be a heartbeat. By now, I would've been able to see it in an ultrasound, moving around. I had so badly wanted to be pregnant, and now, all I wanted was to have this embryo out of me, to move on, to let it go. It was remarkable to me how I reversed the current of my desire.

My doctor recommended a surgical dilation and curettage, which meant that under anesthetic, my uterus's lining would be scraped away and with it, any implanted embryo. It amounted to an abortion. The clinic they recommended was too expensive, costing thousands of dollars, so I went online. Try searching "abortion" on Yelp. There were abortion clinics up near Central Park, as well as Planned Parenthood. In the end, I didn't want to sit with a group of women who didn't want a child. I found a clinic in Chinatown that made oblique mention of pregnancy terminations, and called. The woman who answered told me I could come in the next day.

It turned out this clinic was primarily prenatal, and primarily supporting Chinese and Chinese-American women. I sat in the waiting room with Shahzad, eyeing the bellies around me with numb grief, listening to the conversations in Mandarin and Cantonese. I was asked to approach the front desk, and had to explain what I was there for to a room that fell silent when my sentences unfurled. I clutched a letter from my doctor.

I was taken into another examination room. The doctor was kind, curious. He insisted on doing another ultrasound. Yes, he could see the egg sac. No, he couldn't see a fetal pole (the thickening on the edge of the egg sac that indicates a fetus). Yes, the sac was a lot smaller than it should have been at this stage. No, there was no heartbeat.

He wanted to make sure we understood the whole procedure. We did. Then he decided to describe the process of IVF from the very beginning. It was as if he had forgotten I had already undergone hormone therapy, the extraction of follicular fluid, the fertilization and implantation. If Shahzad and I hadn't known these things at this stage, we would have been remarkably ill-informed, but he said it with such kindness and absurd thoroughness that in exhaustion and nervousness, Shahzad got the giggles. He started to choke with laughter. His only option was to pretend he was crying. The doctor grew more solicitous, which only made it worse. When he left to prepare the operating room, we quietly howled with laughter, crying with relief that we could laugh at this moment, that this was not the worst, that it wasn't even close.

I wanted a local anesthetic, and the doctor insisted on twilight sleep. We went back and forth. The anesthetist was brought in, who also insisted it be twilight sleep. I couldn't work out why they wanted this so badly. Was it because they didn't want to deal with me writhing, or crying? Was it because they'd get more money from my health insurance? The anesthetist's zeal led me to suspect that he was a little bored. Time had passed, and I had to teach in four hours. I gave in.

Ten minutes later I lay back on the operating bed with my legs open, feet propped in stirrups, with the swinging doors opening and shutting to the corridor beyond and patients and nurses casually walking past. I was beyond caring too much. The anesthetist visited and started up small talk, asking me what I wrote about. We ended up talking about art. He had organized an exhibition that was opening in a gallery the following week in Soho. I did a strapped-in double take. "I will ring you with the details," he said. "You'll forget otherwise, with this anesthetic." The IV was in.

I came to twenty minutes later. There was a large glass jar on the counter to the right of the bed filled with blood. They said they would send it away for testing to make sure they got everything. Shahzad and I jumped into the car. Less than half an hour later, I was standing in front of a class of students.

When I woke the next morning, all I felt was relief. It was over.

Had I fallen pregnant naturally—without IVF—I might well not have known it. I have missed periods before. The miscarriage would have been slow to come, but eventually, it would have, and the embryo was small enough for me to not register it as anything other than an ordinary period. All of this only came about because I started looking inside my body, and saw what I didn't consciously know. What had I gained, and what had I lost?

It was tempting to say that the past two months were a waste. I didn't have a pregnancy to show for it—in fact, I'd had my first abortion. My body was still healing from all the needles. I still felt bloated from the hormones. My life was so taken up with the process that I could barely communicate with people outside it. I didn't fault the clinic for my failure; I knew the odds. The overwhelming feeling was that I had rolled the dice, and lost. Two other blastocysts had been frozen. I didn't know if they were abnormal either, though my doctor reassured me that he didn't think they were. He wanted me to register the positive part of the experience. "We know you can get pregnant now," he said. "We know implantation doesn't seem to be a problem." He wanted me to continue. This is what it sounds like to manage your own objectification.

Some people, reading all of this, will see the ways in which the medical industry controlled—to the point of smothering—a pregnancy, and a pregnancy loss. No matter the laughter, or the complications of experience, the outsourcing of conception beyond two bodies is seen as a violence. This suspicion creeps into the most well-reasoned anthropological accounts of IVF. Consider Sarah Franklin's recent analysis of ICSI, the fertilization of an egg by pipette (with sperm inside), and the process that my eggs underwent with Shahzad's sperm. Franklin is probably the most well-known anthropologist today writing about new reproductive technologies, and there are times when her language of close reading persistently assumes the dangers of objectification. She points out how, in videos of the process of ICSI, the egg is, literally, "taken in hand." These videos cannot help but reproduce the point of view of the manipulator and the embryologist, not of the woman. With ICSI, Franklin writes, fertilization is "not narrated as a journey, an adventure romance, or an epic quest, but as a difficult feat of manual control." She suggests we have moved from an act of witness to an act of manipulation, and asks us to consider the consequences. Do we think of that moment of fertilization any differently? After all, our "failure" is all the more visible. Our bodies cannot be left to their own devices, even at a cellular level.

Franklin's interpretation and question sound reasonable, but it's also assumed that it is a violence—in and of itself—to take on the point of view of the embryologist, to internalize it, to absorb a detached view of one's own body. Can't it be *both* an adventure romance and a feat of manual control? Why does it have to be one or the other?

I am aware that I might sound like an apologist for objectification at this point, too much the daughter of a scientist and a doctor, a woman who has so thoroughly internalized an objectifying mode that she can only see the good in it. It's also the case that I could be identifying a neo-Cartesian separation of mind from body that others identify as a broader sign of the times. The philosopher Ian Hacking has pointed out that in the past twenty-five years, multiple forms of medical technology have led us to think of the body as "mere" flesh: we are quite comfortable with organ donation, blood donation, with transplants (both in our own bodies and between bodies), with amputation and genetic splicing, certain that the recombination of body parts or erasure of them does not substantially challenge our sense of integrity of "soul"—or, as he defines it, "character evolved in contact with a world full of people, things, and events." Hacking continues: "We regard our bodies as something other than ourselves, no matter whether we maintain that it is all right to buy and sell body parts, or whether we insist that we can transplant only what has been given freely. In either case, the body is alienated." He might well see the detachment I'm describing as a symptom of a broader bodily alienation that is more contemporary than gendered.

It's also worth pointing out that objectification has never been a particularly stable term, even if it's tempting for writers to treat it that way. In their book *Objectivity*, Lorraine Daston and Peter Galison chart the development of the word from the eighteenth to the twentieth century, identifying three "ages" of objectivity, three ways in which the word was used. They begin with naturalists like Carl Linnaeus and the development of the atlas, which purported to chart the world (and train others to identify things in it). In these atlases, objectivity was a more Platonic truth-to-nature, an analytical ability to "extract the typical from the storehouse of natural particulars"—that is, a convergence of body and mind, sharp and sustained observation, and capacious memory in order to create the most typical representation of a thing. This is the kind of objective impulse that directed early atlases of embryology, or von Baer's drawings, or Leeuwenhoek's accounts of a microscopic world.

With time, some scientists began to understand how flawed this kind of perception could be. To great effect, Daston and Galison describe the experiments in fluid dynamics by Arthur Worthington, who in the nineteenth century had spent years trying to draw by hand the shape of a drop of mercury or milk splashing on a surface. He used a millisecond flash to try to impress on his retina a shape of the liquid just after impact, and drew thousands of images that showed beautifully symmetrical curves and bulges, charting the ways in which the drop widened and separated. In 1894, he began to use photography to improve his process—and was stunned to see how regularly these drops were actually irregularly shaped in the images. When he went back through his years of hand drawings, he realized how consistently he had chosen to overlook these irregularities in his own work. Worthington concluded that in his search for patterns, he had gravitated toward an "ideal splash—an Auto-Splash—whose perfection may never be actually realized." He had been chasing something that didn't exist, all in the name of objectivity.

It was a crushing realization, and it led to a reliance by scientists on devices or scientific methods that would allow them to see without "inference, interpretation, or intelligence." This was, in some sense a "blind sight," and it was directly contrasted to subjectivity as a term. Thus, this second meaning of objectivity moved toward a more automatic sighting. Galison and Daston argued that with the nineteenth century's mania for blind sight, "objectivity" and "subjectivity" took on an oppositional force to one another that actually gave increased force to subjectivity—which, up until that point, had not been a common term to use or worry about. In other words, our awareness of self-perception developed hand in hand with our sense of the non-self, and the two are folded inside one another, even if we treat them as diametrically opposed to one another. To dismiss image-making as an intrinsically objectifying impulse hides the possibility that image-making also invites interpretation, calls it forth.

By the twentieth century, images had become so "blind" they required knowledge to identify them. This was, according to Galison and Daston, when a third interpretation of objectivity developed, which was that of trained judgment. This is the sonographer's eye, measuring a follicle or the width of the uterus. Yes, it is subject to biases. But it would be a mistake to castigate the medical establishment for creating or conferring objectivity as a rule when our epistemological models of seeing turn out to be far more complicated than some analyses would allow.

With the history of the word *objectivity* in mind, the question becomes what kind of "trained judgment" patients are now encouraged to develop. It is easy to look inside ourselves, but harder to know what to do with that knowledge. Having had ICSI performed on my own eggs, I want to consider not just what I lose, but what I gain if I take on the point of view of the embryologist. The visualization of what has, for nearly all time, been a hidden, embodied, often silent and instinctive process, is a remarkable form of self-knowledge. To look inside the body, to understand its constituency, is to understand *more* about the relationship between parts and the whole. Having watched these videos, I am more in awe of the process of conception rather than less. We can understand causality in a new way—perceive, for instance, how infertility is not necessarily mysterious, but the result of a blocked fallopian tube, or endometriosis. Rather than viewing it as a way of removing agency, reproductive technologies could be seen as a way for patients to connect feeling with sight. Initially, it is an awkward mental adjustment, like learning to back up a car for the first time using the rearview mirror. *This* is my body? Ultrasound offers a kind of anatomical recalibration. To emphasize a patient's passivity in the context of a sonogram might also overlook the other emotions she experiences, which is often a rush of joy or feeling when she sees visual confirmation of blood and bone. This can sometimes make her feel more powerful, not less. Not all objectification is surrender; for centuries, portraiture was a way for the wealthy to confirm their power. That their image *could* exist apart from their bodies was a sign of influence in and of itself. To dismiss objectification completely is to miss the pleasure of image-making, which is substantial for those interested in aesthetics in general.

When I remember myself from this time, it is me, standing in front of the mirror, syringe in hand, eyeing my body, gauging my target: a self-portrait of some kind. An adventure romance or journey *is* a feat of manual control.

I had begun the process assuming that waiting was an agony, and it continued to be. But I also started to sense the ways in which the experience was revealing. It had been so easy, up until this point in my life, to not think too hard about the passage of time and my experience of it. I had confidently understood what meaning could be generated in each unit of time: a day, a week, a month, a year. Now, a day could expand like a balloon, and I felt real panic at how neverending each could be. Passing time became a challenge. And yet part of me knew that this panic was important, that I was being presented with a door through which I could understand my life— as in the time I had to live—very differently. It wasn't quite the hyperspace of Mitchison's spacewoman, but it was close. A new way of living had casually revealed itself to me, like the flash of a lining of a coat, visible and crimson.

8

. . .

WORKING GIRL

My mother and I visited New York together for a week when I was thirteen years old. One day, we caught a ferry across to the Statue of Liberty and climbed the staircase inside, looking out through her crown. Copper on the inside, oxidized green on the outside: a gift from France in support of American independence. Even then, it felt like a funny little violation to walk through her. There's a photograph of me posing next to a scale model of her foot in the museum, grinning guiltily, standing over the body of a giant.

Another day, we paid a visit to the Metropolitan Museum and saw a touring exhibition of Honoré Daumier's drawings. I remember being caught by a section devoted to nineteenth-century urban life, particularly his drawings of people on trains: strangers sitting cheek to jowl, all looking off in different directions, companionably moving through space. A boy was asleep, leaning against an older woman. The woman to her right was breastfeeding. In the bench behind, men in black hats spoke among themselves. And here I was, staring at them, feeling far from absentminded about my own movement through space and time. This was the first time I'd encountered an exhibition that I actually liked on my own terms, without obligation or deference to another's choice. I wanted to keep on looking. I remember feeling relieved; I had my own taste! This was a freedom that others would not think to take away; it was such a small thing, this clearing a space in my head. It was a private joy that, as a thirteen-year-old, I had complete control over something.

I was twenty-two when I visited New York City again, this time on a research trip. I was a graduate student and had no money and a friend asked her older sister if I could stay with her. In hindsight, it was extraordinarily generous of the sister to agree. Guests in New York apartments are complicated things. There is never enough room, and you are always stepping to one side, pausing, waiting, for the other to pass by. You hear your guest pissing, flossing, turning over on the couch in the living room. I tried to stay out late and leave early so I wouldn't be a bother, but after the first two nights it was clear she had greater stamina than I; she wasn't home before midnight, and left at five a.m. for the gym. The four-year age difference felt more like ten. She lived a block away from Times Square, hailing distance from a twenty-four-hour neon storm. Her apartment was strikingly modern, with marble counters and the largest and flattest TV screen I had ever seen. I had rarely been in a space before that showed its wealth by its starkness. I marveled at everything; the toiletries in the bathroom, the tiny individual packs of cottage cheese in the fridge (differently flavored), which resembled nutrient packs in a science fiction film. Her lights had *dimmers*. She had a shoe tree. She worked in the financial industry.

I figured out that the gym on the corner offered free week-long trial memberships, and I pretended I was moving to the city. I bought a gym bag, of which I was very proud (it was hefty and square and couldn't be mistaken for anything else) and each evening I used the running machine. It was the first time I had run and watched television at the same time. I watched the other people running to the left and right of me, their absent looks of concentration. They didn't want to look at anyone else. I marveled about how brisk everyone was, buoyed up by the nextness of their lives; they had *this*, then *this*, and after that *this* to do or see.

One night the sister came home early. She took me into her bedroom and opened her built-in wardrobe, where suits hung side by side like skins, and extracted four or five white cotton sacks, which she laid out reverently onto the bed. These, she said, were her bags. She loosened the drawstring on each. Out came a Chanel clutch, a Miu Miu boho, a Prada handbag, and an Yves Saint Laurent tote. I handled each with what I hoped was a suitable amount of care. She told me their prices and that they were an investment. So this is what a young girl's tastes could amount to as well. At the time, I did not notice the clumsy rhyme of my own gym bag. Daumier—known then as a political cartoonist, who had lampooned the rise of the bourgeoisie—would have had a field day with those bags in bags, their nesting emptinesses.

I was spending my twenties living, essentially, hand-to-mouth. My college at Oxford was the wealthiest landowner in the United Kingdom, and I had grown used to the grandeur of the college's quadrangles, its ritualized framing of air and thought, but the stipend I was on barely got me through each month. I lived in rooms that were decorated with the kind of furniture you see in green rooms of regional theaters: nondescript, vaguely woolen, scuffed, scratched, and mismatching. We weren't allowed to take any furniture out of our rooms or put anything in. At Oxford, the scouts—the women who would empty our rubbish bins every day—would inform on you if you did. We ate in the college's dining hall, or cooked in the poorly equipped communal kitchen, where anything beautiful was immediately broken. We didn't think twice about this life, or the fact that all rooms, graduate and undergraduate, were stocked with single beds. It was just one of those things. And so while my friends back home in New Zealand were marrying and having children and buying homes and appointing them with plates and curtains and candles, reading home interior magazines and collecting cookbooks, I experienced a kind of delayed domesticity, studying during the day and getting drunk on cheap liquor at night. I had not yet learned to invest in *things*.

Five years later, when I moved to New York permanently and rented an apartment, the sensation was akin to a hole suddenly appearing in the side of an airplane: that tearing noise, the sudden whoosh of unpressurized air tearing through the cabin. The possibility that I could choose to make my home beautiful took hold. I spent hours on the Ikea website, grew experienced with Craigslist. I began to piece together a history of interior design, and pursued furniture silently, secretively. I wanted it to appear accidental. I began to buy little bowls—at first, cute strange things from Chinatown, then later, from small galleries and design shops. My tastes slowly grew more expensive.

On vacation somewhere, I bought Nancy Meyers's *The Holiday* for $2 on DVD. I had seen her films before, in bits and pieces, on planes and on other people's television sets, not knowing they were made by the same person, and also not knowing they were made by a woman. I had seen Diane Keaton, laughing and crying in a beautiful white office, writing a play. I saw Jack Nicholson grouse his way into her bed. I saw Meryl Streep up a ladder, sparring with Steve Martin. I never remembered any of their characters' names; the actors always appeared to be playing versions of themselves, aggregations of their reputations. *The Holiday* wasn't different. Jude Law and Kate Winslet were charmingly sincere, Jack Black and Cameron Diaz charmingly embarrassing (the Anglo-American cultural switcheroo), but the intrigues were so precisely plotted the whole thing felt a little bloodless. The scenes are snappy, quick: there is no flab. Diaz lives in Los Angeles, Winslet in England. Both are unhappy in love. They swap houses, and each meets a new man. We follow each woman's initial attraction, deepening feeling, complication, and quasi-resolution, all in time for New Year's Eve. With two leading ladies, this is a romantic comedy squared. No wonder it feels as formal as a gavotte. But one night, I accidentally turned on the director's commentary. Ten minutes into the film, Diaz is chucking her boyfriend—who has cheated on her—out of her house. He stands in the courtyard, pleading. Less than ten feet away, the gardener is watering the plants. The boyfriend has to decide whether to explicitly admit his transgression, and he glances over at the gardener—who, very gently, shakes his head. With a sympathetic face and no dialogue, the gardener appears for approximately two seconds in the film before disappearing for good. In her commentary, Meyers noted that they auditioned more than one hundred men for the part.

The weight of this sank in. More than one hundred men for two seconds. This woman knows something, I thought. Or she thinks she knows something. That's when I started watching the film for its backgrounds, ignoring the dialogue or the acting. The interiors of each home—there are remarkably few outdoor scenes in *The Holiday*—are all as precisely judged as the narrative. Diaz's swanky, palatial LA home is shrouded in hibiscus and palms and filled with large lamps and wide couches, whereas Winslet's quaint cottage is shrouded in snow, perched on the outskirts of an English village, and filled with carefully stacked mohair blankets and shabby-chic furniture. (Crate & Barrel vs. Anthropologie.)

All of Meyers's heroines dress in white. They all get to, at some point, triumphantly expel their failed love interest, quite literally, from their house. Their living rooms have comfy, soft linen or cotton sofas—sofas to sink into—which are accompanied by lamps with eggshell linen shades and reclaimed wooden coffee tables. There are tiny, framed prints on the walls, hung in groups like gatherings of swallows. Their kitchens are both well-worn and gleaming, equipped with the finest culinary equipment. Above the Carrara marble counters are open wooden shelves: all the better to display one's thin china bowls on. There are multiple sources of good lighting. Meyers's women laugh a lot. They are financially successful. They drink wine from very large wine glasses. Late at night, Meryl Streep teaches Steve Martin to roll pastry, to make *pain au chocolat*.

In the 1970s, the sociologist Pierre Bourdieu and a team of researchers interviewed thousands of French people about their taste: what they liked to eat, how they liked to exercise, what art they thought interesting. The value of his study—published as the book *Distinction*—lay in how precise his terms were. He measured, for instance, how various career groupings valued the various qualities of their home—among the list, "clean, tidy," "easy to maintain," "practical," "cozy," "comfortable," "warm," "harmonious," "imaginative," and "studied." One career grouping—craftsmen and small business owners—tended to value a home that was clean, tidy, and easy to maintain. Another career grouping—medical services, cultural intermediaries, and art craftsmen—wanted a harmonious, imaginative, and studied home, and they didn't care if it was easy to maintain or not. This is the difference that the prefix of "art" makes. Bourdieu found that people, even at this level of detail, were terribly consistent. He would've found Meyers a wonderful specimen, a kind of Patient Zero for the WASP enthusiasm for all things Parisian.

In the 1990s, a company called Claritas developed a customer segmentation system for marketing in the United States that's referred to as PRIZM, which essentially weaponized findings like Bourdieu's. The PRIZM system categorizes consumers into 14 main groups, based on "urbanicity" and economic class, and further into 68 demographically and behaviorally distinct types or "segments" that help marketers predict a consumer's purchase behavior. The descriptions are horrifying in part because they sound like the beginning of a badly written screenplay. For instance, "Young Digerati" (the fourth group) are described as "the nation's tech-savvy singles and couples living in fashionable neighborhoods on the urban fringe. Affluent, highly educated and ethnically mixed, Young Digerati communities are typically filled with trendy apartments and condos, fitness clubs and clothing boutiques, casual restaurants and all types of bars—from juice to coffee to microbrew." Each group is characterized just as diligently—and all of it circles around what kind of home they want. You have the "Second City Startups," "American Classics," and "Kid Country, USA." There is probably a PRIZM number attached to my Amazon account, to my bank account, to my ZIP code. We like to think there are just three classes— working, middle, upper—but the proliferation of PRIZMs can only mean that consumerism has thrived, its biodiversity exploded. They show you just how complicated the notion of the middle class in the United States has become, and how aspirational it always is.

Once you've read about these PRIZM segments, it's hard to avoid seeing them in operation everywhere. For example: Mike Nichols's film *Working Girl* (1988) is a classic rags-to-riches story about a working-class girl making good in the Big Apple, but it is not just about the move from *petite* to *haute*: Tess (played by Melanie Griffith) wants to move from group no. 40, "Aspiring A-Lister" ("Typically urban renters, aspiring A-Listers are focused on their social lives") to group no. 7, "Money and Brains," who have "high incomes, advanced degrees, and sophisticated tastes to match their credentials." Tess achieves this by attempting to impersonate Katharine, her WASPy boss (played by Sigourney Weaver). The emotional force of the film comes from how precisely it charts class. We watch Tess transform her hair, jewelry, lingerie, clothes, accent.

The most interesting thing about the movie is that though Tess changes a lot about herself, her business acumen remains qualitatively different from her boss's. She anticipates the market based on her reading of dailies and gossip magazines rather than the *Wall Street Journal*, using social composites of PRIZMs before they were even articulated. She's a bellwether for the power of micro–consumer purchases, a new kind of woman on Wall Street, with, as she says drunkenly, "a head for business and a bod for sin." It's implied, ever so slightly, that her head is this way *because* of her bod—or at least, the ways she has learned to look after her body have led her to think this way about business. The film indirectly argues that a woman's femininity is defined by her economic privilege, and proposes the reverse could be true: that her privilege could be changed by how she expresses her femininity. It is not a comfortable equation to consider.

For a long time, I did not want to accept the crude reductive force of PRIZM, or of the suggestion that my economic privilege directed how I performed being a woman. I thought I could get away with avoiding it; I did not "take care of myself" in the way either Tess or Katharine did. But that's a PRIZM too. I was slow on the uptake: this is also what a woman's taste amounts to. And so when I turned to consider IVF, I was also slow to realize that my understanding of fertility and how to fix it was also a micro–consumer purchase. You could categorize people and their reproductive choices into 68 behaviorally distinct segments: I'm sure that in some blue-mirrored building in Virginia, it has been done. How I decorate my home is connected to how I address my fertility. Worse than that: one *predicts* the other. This is why Meyers's films are so fascinating to watch: she understands how domestic space structures her characters. It is a claustrophobic connectivity. Art is not exempt from a gestalt so fundamentally defined by capitalism. My love for Daumier felt like a reprieve, but it is too easily transformed into a form of currency. IVF had felt like a rupture in my life, but my reproductive failure had already been anticipated, a plot twist in a badly written screenplay. No. 69, "Career gal who's left it till too late." This is what a woman's taste amounts to. Indeed, it's remarkably easy to invent more about motherhood. No. 70, "Artificial intelligence: games designed to build the infant brain." No. 71, "Gender-neutral everything." No. 72, "None of her friends are mothers." No. 73, "All her friends are mothers."

These hypothetical PRIZMs might sound silly until you visit a playground and notice how a mother—particularly with her first child—is forced to make a series of choices about "basic" objects (strollers, Tupperware, diapers, clothes, shoes, games) that market themselves according to what kind of mother a woman wants to be. It's her choice, of course—but her choices direct her, too, nudge her one way or another. Bourdieu's distinction has an uncanny predictive force for babies. Do you want a baby that is clean, tidy, and easy to maintain? Or do you want a baby that is harmonious, imaginative, and studied, and you don't care if it is easy to maintain or not? Do you want a nanny who is from another class to temper your own habits, to course-correct your child out of one PRIZM and into another? How a woman clothes her body after birth—what she hides and does not hide, how she expresses her sexuality as available or not—all adds up to a public expression of self.

If you think I am reaching here, think of the obsessiveness with which people online—mostly ciswomen—share pictures of the nurseries they have decorated in anticipation of their child: the exact paint color, the crib, the various images and boxes and changing tables. Think of the baby shower, the almost physical compulsion some people feel to buy a gift for an infant when it arrives. Most of us have a memory, even if it's fake, of exhausted new mothers and fathers discussing the merits of various models of a *thing*; we don't even have to know if it is a stroller or type of feeding bottle. We imagine their rising and falling tones, the cadence of their microdistinctions: playground shoptalk. In this country, aesthetic taste has been so tightly tied to spending power, has been expressed so pervasively in the form of the domestic, in the well-appointed home, that it is very hard for the abstract thought of a child to *not* also be an expression of economic privilege. Babies become objects *because* they are costly. This is what a mother's taste might amount to.

In 1980, the French theorist Roland Barthes published *Camera*

Lucida, a short, moving, and maddening book about photography that argued that images could contain, among other things, the elements of *studium* and *punctum*. This theory was his way of arguing why some images moved us more than others. *Studium* referred to "a classical body of information": what we expect a photograph of that subject to contain. It offered "a kind of general, enthusiastic commitment," "that very wide field of unconcerned desire, of various interest, of inconsequential taste: *I like / I don't like*." For Barthes, the *studium* was "of the order of liking, not of loving"; it mobilized a "half desire, a demi-volition; it is the same sort of vague, slippery, irresponsible interest one takes in the people, the entertainments, the books, the clothes one finds 'all right.'" It was *punctum* that moved Barthes, that "punctuated" the *studium*—"this element which rises from the scene, shoots out of it like an arrow, and pierces me." The details of a photograph that moved Barthes, that made it poignant to him, that bruised him, reminded him of the mortality of the object in the image, the remorselessness of time.

As aesthetic theories go, it's alluringly transposable. Although Barthes dismissed *studium*, he did a good enough job defining it for us to see that "half desire" in other areas. PRIZMs are *studium*. The living rooms in Meyers's films appear as exercises in a *studium* of the domestic, maneuvers in taste, subject to quiet ecstasies of approval. They belong to the order of liking, not loving. Nobody wants to say they *love* their sofa; that is, the way that you love a person, all in, unevenly, grandly. And in the early twenty-first century, motherhood—or at least, the framing of it—seems to be an exercise in *studium*, too, despite the fact that it is literally an exercise in being punctured. Giving birth is one of the few occasions where women feel entitled to publicly describe the intensity of a wound, but the pain, the disorientation and bruising, is rarely lingered on. If it is, it is firmly bracketed in the narrative of birth, extolled as "natural," and what women are encouraged to move on to, very quickly, is a *studium* of the domestic: a successful parent is one who has everything under control, who can serenely move through life, calmly doing three things at once, meeting their child's bellowing tantrum with quiet reason, not nagging or scolding, finding time for body and mind, completing an endless succession of facile tasks with a kind of domestic *sprezzatura*.

IVF follows in lockstep. The rhetoric of new reproductive technologies on brochures in waiting rooms are bodies of information that frantically try to contain suffering. The waiting room with its inoffensive abstract art, lamps and magazines and upholstered chairs is designed to remind you, ever so gently, that even domestic spaces can be public ones. You cannot be vulnerable, even if your comfort is provided for. Ushered into a cubicle to give blood, you are very aware of the five or so other women sitting next to you, in other cubicles, each attended to by a nurse. It would not do to make a fuss. You watch the nurse's face as she concentrates on finding a vein, then inserts the needle. Every morning she draws blood, which means she could possibly see a hundred women a day. If she has worked here for a few years, she will have taken blood from tens of thousands of women by now. She has a remarkably warm smile, but you barely speak. What can you say? There doesn't seem to be time. There never is. You are always waiting to be seen—examined swiftly—then it is back to waiting some more. Results are always after the fact. The experience is akin to stroking a cat with such quiet force that it is compelled to stay lying down. Pain is always to be managed, and if it is to be actually experienced, there is the expectation that this will be done in private. The ultimate compliment is that the procedure "went smoothly."

If you think that this is just a function of the medical sphere, I would point out that the message boards, with their coy acronyms and stork emoji, also anticipate and corral pain. IVF anticipates the general tone of motherhood before you are even pregnant because it anticipates, even mimics, the notion of justified pain—the despair of sustained sleeplessness, of a child that punches you in the eye because you are trying to stop them from falling in the river, the endlessness of the work involved. What I find remarkable is how *little* has changed with IVF. This is how J. B. S. Haldane described the hypothetical "procedure" that women underwent to remove their wombs in his pamphlet "Daedalus" in 1924: the operation, he predicted, was "somewhat unpleasant, though now no longer disfiguring or dangerous, and never physiologically injurious, and is therefore an honour but by no means a pleasure." The qualifications in this sentence, the seeming necessity of each slight adjustment, the parsing between honor and pleasure, the defensiveness and exactitude—I can think of no sentence that better enacts the balancing act of assisted reproductive technologies in the twentieth and twenty-first centuries.

9

. . .

AT NORTH FARM

The second time through IVF was more *studium*, less *punctum*. The imposition of needles and routines felt more manageable. I didn't burst into tears. I grew comfortable ducking routine questions about my life. I didn't return to the acupuncturist in midtown; I didn't have time. The first time was in summer, when work was slow, but now it was autumn, and I was in the middle of a busy semester. My reading of the message boards tapered off; I felt like I had learned nearly every story there, and now it was just the pain of repetition. In the waiting room, I was able to read my book, rather than look at the women. More follicles, more crosshairs. I could've used one of the frozen blastocysts, but the doctor told me that if I wanted a sibling, it was better to do it again now than try in a couple of years. What strikes me now is how little I hesitated doing it all over again. I ordered more hormones. My body was constantly bruised, constantly healing from the injections. The second operation, Shahzad was there to pick me up. ICSI again. For whatever reason—hormones, stimulation protocols, stress, the lack of tea, and acupuncture—the embryos this time around were fewer, and less robust. There were three of them. Rather than wait five days, until they could become blastocysts, they decided to implant them at three days. One, the embryologist said, looked really good. He gave me another picture. I did not put this one on the mantelpiece; I knew better. I hid it away in a book, until I knew.

The night before my pregnancy blood test, I came home from seeing a film, giddy with the news that I'd been awarded a six-month writing residency back in New Zealand, which was to begin the following July. They'd rung me in the lobby of the theatre, and I felt the rare vertigo that comes when you feel your life changing right in front of your eyes. I wondered what else might change as swiftly. At the pharmacy next to the subway station, I bought a pregnancy test, and back home, peed on the stick. Five minutes later. A horizontal and a vertical line: a window. I was stunned. I had felt absolutely nothing: no implantation cramps, thirstiness, or nausea, no swollen breasts.

I knew to constrain my excitement. I would have to wait: wait for an appropriate set of hCG blood results, wait until eight weeks (when the chance of miscarriage fell a significant percent), then to thirteen weeks (for the first round of fetal testing), and then onward through every testing and developmental milestone, to nine months. I was not out of the woods. I was never going to be out of the woods until I had a baby in my arms. I rang my father. I told him the good news about the residency and the pregnancy. "Oh, Jenni," he said, and I could hear the pain in his voice. "You'll have to give up the residency." I did not give myself the chance to either grieve his accuracy (the residency rescinded their offer once I told them), or resent his sorrow.

To my surprise, nothing terrible happened. At six weeks, I saw the heartbeat, strong and fast. It felt deeply odd to see and hear the sound, and not know the truth of it from my body. Nausea came and went, and when it did pass, I immediately started to worry it was a sign of an impending miscarriage. Still nothing. I was officially "transferred" from my IVF clinic to an ob/gyn. I went on another writing residency, this time to New Hampshire, for a month in the depths of winter. I drove to and from the hospital for my NIPT—a major milestone in terms of chromosomal abnormalities, and one which predicts the sex—and one night, alone in the library, the dark pressing in, opened the email of my test results. The fetus was female. I looked up at the empty room, grinning. I had told no one there I was pregnant, for fear they would not let me walk the icy roads to the cabin they'd given me, a mile away, deep in the woods. I set off, holding my flashlight, wearing my snow grippers, listening to the snow shifting in the tree branches, the occasional movement in the trees beyond. I was going to have a girl.

I was closer to inhabiting a fairy tale than I had ever been. For lunch, they literally delivered a wicker basket of food to my cabin door. I kept on expecting a voice to issue forth from the trees, or for strange footprints to appear on the snowy path. I started rereading Angela Carter's short stories, which I had fallen in love with as a fourteen-year-old. Carter is probably most well known for her reformulations of fairy tales—"Beauty and the Beast," "Bluebeard," "Peter and the Wolf," "Puss-In-Boots"—that rewrite our sense of moral consequence. Many of her narrators are young women, aware of their inexperience, but they do not shrink from death or dissolution. Beauty *wants* to be devoured. Part of the pleasure in reading Carter comes from seeing how she rewires the moral calculus of stories you already knew. Quite naturally, I started to think about questions of inheritance. What fairytales would I tell my child? What would she need to know? I was carrying a chalice, a letter, a package of coins for someone else. Every third day, I drove to a local mountain and climbed my way up it, feeling the cold air in my lungs, the blood rushing through my body, concentrating on the choreography of my legs and arms as I climbed. At the center of me was a thing not me, rapidly expanding.

Though I was supposed to spend each night in a shared house close to the dining hall, I far preferred sleeping in the cabin that had been assigned to me for writing during the day. I was testing my fear; it was one of the few times I could remember regularly sleeping almost a mile away from any other human being, with no car, no cell phone or Wi-Fi service. I would lie there at night, listening to the creaking radiator, the stillness outside, and concentrate on her inside me, curled up. I had taken to calling her the bean. If any beast arrived, we were on our own. If I told anyone—my friends, my mother—I immediately reminded them how swiftly it could all end.

Motherhood felt abstract because it was aspirational and because my family lived half a world away and because virtually none of my friends in New York City had kids. The internet became my atlas, my way of knowing, and the fact that it was constructed by others' prior searches was both comforting and terrifying. At first I thought it was a collective id of pregnancy, but the more I looked, the more it all seemed less id and more superego: this is what it always was, and therefore should be. If you type "pregnancy" into Google Image search, you are presented with a sea of bellies, all six or seven months along—big enough to definitively show that clear swell, the confident burst of flesh, but not so big that your first thought is to flinch. Around 95 percent of the images are of white bellies. More often than not, you do not see the mother's face; she is either cropped out, or she is looking away, either to refuse our gaze or to hide her face. Her hands are often more important; they hold the belly, one at the top, the other at the bottom, framing the screen of flesh, telling us where to look: a tiny movie screen. Inside, there is life. These images were so strikingly consistent they appeared archetypal, vehicles for desire that was also a fullness, a profound satiation. If you typed in a specific week of pregnancy, you were confronted by thousands of images of women who had posted photos of their baby bumps. This is what 16 weeks looks like on one body. This is what 32 does on another. They pose side-on, excited and alarmed, in front of chalkboards and poster paper that list fun facts. They were generally white, and often dressed in yoga gear. They had to-do lists and couldn't wait to meet their little one. I did not realize you could be this upbeat and organized about pregnancy until the internet taught me.

There were hundreds of websites giving me updates on my fetus's development. She was as big as a blueberry, cherry, apricot, melon. She had fingerprints. She was hiccupping. She was learning to swallow, to open her eyes, to clench and unclench her fingers. She was learning how to suck, to latch, to breathe. She could recognize my voice over the pounding of my heart and the rushing of my organs, which must sound like the incessant white noise of a plane's cabin. The illustrations of fetuses were inevitably done in soft shades of pink. They floated very calmly in space. They did not thrash or tumble, were not squished or covered in goo, were not fish-like or primate-like, and did not remind you of anything other than a baby, cleaned and camera ready. I did not know what to do with any of these images, all exercises in *studium* rather than *punctum*.

So I barely took any photos, let alone with a chalkboard. This could've been a deliberate resistance, or because I was so fearful of losing her, or both. I did not buy anything for her. It wasn't until I was 22 weeks along (quite clearly showing) that I actually felt her move one night, back in New York, as I was lying in bed: a gentle tickle deep in my pelvis. It took a few more nights before I was confident enough to name this as *her* rather than indigestion. And still I said nothing, barely, to anyone. I did not call her my "daughter," or use the word "mother." I couldn't say "baby" or "child." I found it hard to parse the difference between paranoia and superstition. All those women in fairy tales who had hoped and prayed for a child, and then what happened? I was afraid any presumption of mine would be punished by some force in which I did not even believe. I kept on waiting for the cat-mother-gut wisdom that so many women talked about to show up, but it never really did.

During these months, the beginning of John Ashbery's poem "At North Farm" wouldn't leave me alone; I'd be walking along, and suddenly realize I was silently chanting it.

> Somewhere someone is traveling furiously toward you,
> At incredible speed, traveling day and night,
> Through blizzards and desert heat, across torrents,
>   through narrow passes.
> But will he know where to find you,
> Recognize you when he sees you,
> Give you the thing he has for you?

This baby was a long-awaited stranger, a relative I had never met. As she grew bigger, I started to see her movements beneath my skin; my stomach would look visibly lopsided when she settled to the right or the left. Sometimes she moved in two different directions, stretching her legs and arms or head, arching her back—and everything on the surface twisted, like a cloth being wrung out, or a wave deep in the ocean, far from shore. She moved in me as people do in bed, sleeping, strangely intent on a world even further in, her universe swiftly expanding, my own body pushing outward. I bought two black dresses and one jumpsuit and wore them over and over again: my pregnancy uniform.

When I was seven months along, I stayed at a friend's for a night and woke in the morning to a string of text messages and missed calls: at around two a. m., the apartment above mine in my building had caught fire, and the fire department had sent vast quantities of water through the building to put it out, wrecking the kitchens and bathrooms on five floors, including mine. There was asbestos and smoke in the air. It wasn't safe to return home; I was allowed into my apartment for ten minutes to pack a bag. The entire place was up-ended, fragmented, sodden; you couldn't think or talk over the industrial dehumidifiers set up everywhere. Shahzad was touring in Europe.

I found it bizarrely appropriate. Of course I wouldn't plan for a nursery. Of course I wouldn't *nest*. Another friend kindly offered me her apartment in the East Village that she was waiting for co-op approval to renovate. It had no real kitchen, no furniture to speak of other than a blow-up mattress, but it had walls and windows and a shower and a toilet, and an amazing view, out over Alphabet City and the East River beyond. For the last two months of my pregnancy, I woke before dawn to the sounds of doves, and watched the pink sunlight grow and swell along the brick walls. It grew hot. I strode along the street on clogs, swollen to the point that people I passed would visibly wince, and I went to as many movies as I could to take advantage of their air conditioning. Her heartbeat was eerily regular at my weekly appointments at the hospital, and the nurse had to poke my stomach repeatedly to get her to move. She was in her own time zone. In the hospital, I drank cold water and listened to the amplified thwack of her heart in the room, the jostling noises as she turned left or right. I felt alone in my situation, and part of me knew to enjoy it. I met my doula, Stephanie, went to work, met friends, and waited for her to hatch.

I was asked to develop a "birthing plan" for any medical staff I'd see when admitted, which felt both useful and useless. On the one hand, I learned about how pain relief made it harder to push, which in turn increased the chances of a cesarean, which in turn increased the recovery time. A natural birth offered the best outcome for me and a baby. But I found it ludicrous to print out these expectations when it was also obvious that everything could and would change in an instant. The plan looked comical to me, as naive as a child's list for Santa, and I feared that I would only feel like a failure when I inevitably departed from it.

My due date came and went. One day, two days. Three days. She showed no sign of descending or arriving. I had organized my working life to neatly come to a pause when she was due, and now the clock was ticking on the time I had off to be with her. I had not thought about having to wait *more*. Shahzad returned and we moved into a six-week sublet together. At four in the morning on the fifth day, I woke to feel my insides pulling in and twisting quite convulsively, but also quite bearably. The movement was reflexive in the same way an orgasm is; you cannot help but let go. I had breakfast with a friend, went for a walk, sat in a terrible café reading a good novel. But toward the evening and after a second walk, the contractions became closer together, and more painful. They developed peaks and valleys of intensity, and at their height, I began to moan involuntarily from the pain. By ten in the evening, as I lay on the sofa, it hurt enough that each time, I started to instinctively reach my arm up to the sky, as if grabbing for a rope that would pull me out of my body. I called Stephanie. Three hours later, as the three of us drove to the hospital, I was groaning constantly, hanging over the back seat, looking at the empty Manhattan Bridge receding behind me. My vision was slowly closing down: by the time we made it into the hot tub at the hospital's birthing center, I opened my eyes only for brief moments, could not stand or sit, and had devolved to a crouch, slow rocking motions, and loud groaning. I did not think about the fact that all of these movements and behaviors were those of an infant.

Though there was no point in opening my eyes or talking, it was absurdly comforting to hold Shahzad's and Stephanie's hands. I lost track of many things, but I knew whose hand was which, and that I was not alone. I don't think I let go of more than one hand for about nine hours.

Every so often, the midwives would inspect my cervix to see how much it had dilated, and when they did, I could feel hands wiping liquids away from me. They spotted dark green meconium (her feces), which indicated she was in distress, and announced they were moving me upstairs, to the delivery floor, where they had me lie down, inserted an IV into my arm, and started a constant monitoring of her heartbeat. The midwife disappeared: another birth, complicated, a cesarean. I nodded, eyes closed.

By five a.m., the terror was not in the pain of one convulsion, but in the knowledge that I would have to do this for an unspecified period of time. I began to shake uncontrollably. My contractions were about a minute apart, and had been that way for hours. As each one arrived, I would moan and writhe, holding on to the bars of the bed with such force that my arms ached for days afterward. Her heartbeat was increasing, and Shahzad kept telling me to slow her heart by slowing mine. Breathe deeply in, and out, he said, over and over again. We listened to hers slow—then I would forget, and everything would speed up again. He fell asleep, midmantra, exhausted, and I gripped Stephanie's hand, terrified. I asked about an epidural. It was too late for that, they said.

Looking back, I cannot resurrect the actual sensation of the pain. Though my eyes stayed closed, I can construct the image of my body on the bed. I remember thinking that this was the closest I was going to come to dying before death itself. I was skating close to the cessation of consciousness.

At seven-thirty, they told me that it was time to push. I had not reflected on what it would feel like to lie on your back, bend and open your legs as wide as they could go, and be asked to hold on to the back of your own thighs—in other words, to be primarily responsible for a humiliating vulnerability. (There is a very similar yoga pose called Happy Baby, which now seems like a very bad joke.) Multiple people hovered over me, chanting, cheering me on. Decades of bladder control and social training were pushed aside with one brusque shove. With each contraction, I squeezed with all my energy. "Harder!" they cried. "Harder!" I could not go harder. I felt flesh tearing. It didn't feel right or natural to hurt myself that way; the sensation was akin to trying to break one arm with the other.

And then it happened very quickly—a slithering feeling that could have been a noise or a sensation, a long string of something passing through me, and they called for me to open my eyes. "You have a baby," they said. "You did it." They took her away immediately to aspirate her, to remove the meconium from her mouth and nose, but she was yelling before they even reached the table. I saw her gray body being carried aloft, all head and a long torso like a tadpole, and I thought, *That is a baby. That is my baby.* It was nine a.m.

They cleaned her up before giving her to me. I wished I had seen her as she was inside me, covered in my liquids. They had put a little hat on her. She snuffled at my breastbone, smelled milk, but within a minute, fell asleep, exhausted. I looked at her face. It was true that I did not recognize her. I could not stop looking at her, trying to engrave her face in my neural cortex. While all of this was happening I birthed the placenta, which simply felt like a mass of material moving through me. Then the midwife began to stitch me up. I could feel pain from the needle passing through me, the tug of the thread against my skin, but it felt like nothing next to what had come before.

Shahzad held the computer over my bed, allowed my own mother to see me, lying there, with my baby. I did not understand then the relief she must have felt—to know that I had passed through the forest, had emerged, in the sunlight, on the other side. I allowed myself, for the first time, to call this child by her name. Anika.

In the recovery ward, my nurse, Gigi, held Anika in her arms and led me to the bathroom, and told me I needed to pee. My body was so confused, I couldn't isolate the right muscles with my mind. In the end, I had to use a squeeze bottle to squirt water on my labia—and only then, in a sympathetic response, I urinated. I was told to use a pain relief spray that settled like a white dusting of snow. Gigi explained how to assemble a pad to absorb all of the blood I was about to expel from my body. It was the sanitary pad system to end all menstrual events, a battleship composed of disposable mesh panties, a liner sheet folded in half, three fat menstrual pads, and witch-hazel circles of cloth that soothe and cool. Climbing back up on the bed took real effort. I felt beaten up. It was only when eating my first solid food since the labor had begun that I started to realize I had passed through the eye of the needle. I had survived. Being fit and strong, I had not realized it would be such a debatable matter. Any euphoria came from pure relief. I was still seeing double from tiredness. Anika would wake—her dark eyes regarding me, pulling to focus—then fall back asleep again. Gigi held my breast, molding it, showing me how to direct the nipple into her mouth. When she began to suck, it felt like she was pulling on strings anchored deep within me. I felt intensely grateful for Gigi, and asked her question after question. How do you burp? How do you hold the head up? How warm does she need to be? How does this car seat work? She patiently answered each question. At night, they came to take Anika from me for a few hours. I could not understand how she would be OK away from me. It was the first time she was out of reach. I also cried with relief. This baby required everything, all the time, and that day, I felt my past life being taken away as smoothly and efficiently as the nurses took her that evening. In the lactation class the next morning, I sat next to six women, all first-time parents, our babies in Plexiglas bassinets at our sides. Our progeny lay beside us, caught fish, occasionally twitching, going nowhere. The consultant squeezed a knitted woolen breast she had bought on Etsy, and we leaned forward, trying to learn.

Two days later, I walked, slowly, up the road to buy tacos. I was still bleeding, and would bleed for a month more. Whole pieces of tissue had already emerged. I marveled that no one seemed to notice. My breasts were hard with milk. I was disintegrating, piece by piece, back toward my old body, the cells absorbing what they could, sending the rest out into space. I could not stop the liquids seeping, could not hold myself back, draw a distinction between myself and the world around me. My empty stomach jostled with each movement. Anika was against my chest. I was still learning to hold her, trying to gauge the bobbing weight of her head against my hand. I was spending all day and night trying to pour myself into her. On the couch, her little jaw worked furiously as she took in the milk. We were two characters spinning through space, living far beyond the civilization of my life before. When she slept, she sometimes shivered, trembled as if she was dreaming: her own internal big bang receding, receding, in her mind. I cleaned her of fluids, gave her new ones, and learned to live with the nightmare of dissolving boundaries.

Other people arrived to look at her and me. I had no idea what to say to them: I had barely any idea of what to say to myself. One vast wave of baby desiring had given way to another equally vast swell of baby growing, and my psyche could not catch up. I was functioning: talking to insurance companies, working out a bridging loan, putting in an offer on a new apartment. I kept clean. I dealt with the nightmare of very little breast milk, which involved feeding Anika, then pumping—in order to increase my supply—every two hours, twenty-four hours a day. My nipples bled, they were so overworked; at times, Anika was drinking pink milk. I walked to the park most days. I didn't really sleep. A seemingly endless supply of adrenaline seemed to move through my body. There was so much to learn: how to use a sling, how to use a breast pump, how to use a car seat. I was forever reading manuals. But I still could not call myself a mother, and could barely bring myself to push a stroller. I felt like an impostor. I kept on looking at Anika's face, worried that I was not learning it quickly enough, worried I could not tell her cry from others'.

Years later, when reading Charis Thompson's book *Making Parents*, I winced when she described women who'd undergone IVF who would not allow themselves to enjoy their pregnancy, who were always waiting for the axe to fall, who could barely understand themselves as mothers when their children were born: who had managed their infertility so carefully that they didn't know what to do with their fertility. I can see the truth of that in me. Throughout the pregnancy, I fought like hell to be happy, to be calm, to not allow the experience to overwhelm me, but I was as far from "blithe" as could be. When I recall this time, I notice how I moved into, from the day of my first IVF appointment, a series of nested exhaustions—the exhaustion of diagnosis, of stimulation, of operation, of waiting—and how these exhaustions continued beyond IVF, into pregnancy, birth, and into looking after an infant. It's easy to think of them in series, and because you do, even to anticipate whatever the next experience will be as another exhaustion. In my case, with a largely uneventful pregnancy and birth, the exhaustion came mostly from fear. Pregnancy did not make me feel more female: it made me feel more mortal.

But this anxiety was also because I did not want to be a PRIZM of motherhood. I was keenly aware that in the absence of a community I loved that showed me how to be a mother, marketing might well creep into the gap. I was caught between advice and accoutrement, unsure of what it meant to navigate all that I did not know by purchasing wisdom: a breastfeeding consultation, a white noise machine, diaper cream.

I could've dismissed the expectation to *enjoy* a pregnancy as unnecessarily limiting. I could've focused, instead, on the way time continued to do funny things. For almost a year, my life had been strictly divided up into weeks—the rhythm of my appointments depended on it—but now that I could not sleep for more than two or three hours at a time, the days took on a hallucinogenic length. I would read at three a.m., watch movies at eight a.m., bake a cake at midnight. The weeks seemed laughably arbitrary. I lost track of what day it was.

I could have also paid attention to the growing knowledge of myself as an animal, as having an animal's body that inhaled and exhaled, and ate and excreted. When I was pregnant, I felt it most clearly in bed, in the moments before and after sleep: in other words, in plain sight of my tiredness. I would feel my body resting, pausing, and understand what a pleasure it was to simply lie there, alive, and watch the light shift in patterns on the wall. The quietness of my existence was the best part of it. Once Anika was born, the only pauses were in the moments she fed or slept, which felt unbearably brief for all the time I spent trying to *get* her to feed or sleep. The knowing I sensed pregnant was the same, refracted, intensified once she was born: it came from watching her as an animal, feeling her stillness, her eyes tracking the light, her weight asleep, the sound of her breath. The knowing was being able to witness, feel, her living body. I didn't want to read a book about it, or read an online article. All I really wanted to do was watch online videos of gorillas with their infants. The mothers would look away, almost ostentatiously casual, but their arms moved so swiftly when their child stumbled. Their alert looseness was educational as I learned my own grip. I said none of this to friends. When other adults looked at her face, I heard the same phrase over and over again. *Look how innocent she is.* I couldn't get my head around what they were seeing. Yes, she knew nothing of elections, stabbings, and Olympic gymnastic competitions; she did not know how to control her own limbs, could barely lift her own head up. But I could see how much other knowledge she already had. She knew how to breathe through her nose and feed with her mouth, how to sneeze or hiccup. If she choked on my milk, she knew how to cough it up. I would trace her skull and examine the faint blue veins beneath the skin. My body had knitted the most intricate creature together. Her complexity utterly and completely exceeded my consciousness. Innocence seemed quaintly biblical, a worn-out moral. It wasn't something to lose, like a toy, but something that might grow or wither. I sat looking down at her, and Anika would stare back up at me, growing recognition in her eyes—of me, but also of life, of what it was like to be an animal in this world of light.

10

THE WALKING EGG

When Anika was three months old, Shahzad and I traveled with her to Europe. Our first stop was Britain, to visit Bourn Hall, the world's first IVF clinic, which was established by Robert Edwards, Patrick Steptoe, and Jean Purdy in 1980.

Bourn Hall was barely eight miles from Cambridge; Purdy, searching through real estate listings, had found the Jacobean manor house, which included a chapel, stables, and outbuildings, all on twenty acres of parkland. The property had passed through many hands; the site of an eleventh-century moated castle, it had been destroyed during the Barons' Wars in the thirteenth century, then rebuilt and modified by several generations of owners. The *Daily Mail*, remarkably, purchased the estate for Edwards and Steptoe in 1979, then pulled out; they thought the venture "too risky." Edwards and Steptoe had to raise the capital elsewhere, through the combination of private investors and foundations. Bourn Hall first opened its doors to twenty-three women in September 1980.

Our drive from London—the endless number of roundabouts, the pub lunch, the small villages we wound our way through—felt achingly familiar to me, as did Bourn Hall: having spent all that time at Oxford, I recognized the look and smell of upper-class institutional: the slightly shabby carpet, the odd proportions of rooms, the repurposing of a building for a slightly different kind of privilege. It was a grand house, but a composite one, a patchwork of embellishment. In the conference room, wood carvings from different centuries were incorporated into the dark wooden walls, and the fireplace molding was part of a four-poster bed from a demolished estate nearby. This used to be Steptoe's office. We sat around a large table. They had arranged a series of meetings for me: with the director, with the head embryologist, with the clinic manager. Their publicist politely hovered. I had assumed they would want to hide Shahzad and Anika away in a spare office while I spoke with them; in my own IVF clinic in New York, children were not allowed in the waiting room. But they waved them both on to the dining room, and gave Shahzad some free coffee tokens. Their presence turned out to be relaxing. Somehow, everyone knew Anika was an IVF baby. I was, ideologically speaking, part of the family.

In the early years of the clinic, patients needed to live on the grounds for approximately two weeks at a stretch. Edwards, Steptoe, and Purdy erected plywood portacabins to house them (along with clinical, operating, and laboratory facilities), and in the morning, the women walked from their cabins to the main house, across the grass, in their dressing gowns. In the dining room where Shahzad and Anika now were, the women ate alongside the doctors and staff; two chefs cooked all the meals. During the day, patients amused themselves with board games and television. Outside, there were sun chairs and a pitch and putt set. Steptoe would occasionally play the piano. There was a prayer room. Husbands were not allowed to stay with their wives, and so the men took rooms in the dozens of bed-and-breakfasts that sprung up around Bourn Hall, playing pool and drinking together down at the local pub. There were visiting hours. No children were allowed. Very few couples actually told their families and friends where they were and what they were doing. Instead, they simply went on "holiday." The setup was a far cry from Huxley's Central London Hatchery and Conditioning Centre, but even if it undersold notions of medical and clinical efficiency, it enacted the normalizing traditions of upward class mobility: posh, but not too posh. The evocation of class probably helped manage any fears about the radical quality of IVF, or its sense of experimentation.

Accounts of the clinic's early routine have a lenticular quality: tilt them one way, and they appear almost defiantly normalizing; tilt them another, and they seem as socially experimental as Mitchison's *Memoirs of a Spacewoman*. In the beginning, none of the patients were undergoing hormonal stimulation, and so their urine had to be religiously collected and tested to detect rising progesterone and estrogen levels and predict their ovulation. Women were expected to carry a plastic jug around with them at all times to pee into, and every morning, take the previous twenty-four hours' worth of urine to the endocrinology lab for testing. It wasn't uncommon to see a group of women taking a walk to the nearby village, each with a jug in hand, seemingly determined to accommodate the awkward realities of their situation. Ann Hartley, who was a patient in 1981, remembered her time there as inescapably social: the women had little to do but talk to each other, discussing their cycles and egg retrievals. Operations, timed to coincide with naturally occurring ovulations, happened at every hour of the day and night. Once the embryo was implanted, they were expected to lie down for three days. Everyone knew when someone was waiting to find out if an implantation had worked. When she disappeared abruptly, without celebration, it was clear what had happened. Hartley recalled around thirty women in residence. (Within a year, the clinic was treating sixty women a month.) The success rate was around 10 percent. Hartley was the only one of the women who were treated alongside her to fall pregnant.

Hartley was referred to Bourn Hall through the National Health Service, but most patients paid the £1,800 fee (about £9,000 today), almost a third of the then–national average salary of £6,000. The range in fee structure made for a heterogeneous group of women. In the 1980s and 1990s, the Icelandic government paid for a group of women to visit Bourn Hall each year—the staff called them the "dottirs" (after the Icelandic suffix for "daughter" attached to a patronymic). One year their visit coincided with Iceland's day of national independence, and the entire group walked up the long driveway waving the national flag. Other heterogeneities were harder to nostalgically recuperate. There were foreign wives of businessmen who turned up, for whom translators were arranged—only to discover that they did not know why they were being sent to Bourn Hall, or what was about to happen. A few times, the same husband would return a second time with a different wife, even if his infertility was quite possibly the issue.

Edwards and Steptoe were notoriously casual about their finances. They had gone into business almost without meaning to at the ages of fifty-eight and seventy-one respectively, and the whole notion of a "bottom line" seemed a secondary consideration. (Bourn Hall would go bankrupt in the late 1980s, and avoided closure when it was bought by the pharmaceutical company Serono, the same company that produced Pergonal. The clinic was able to purchase itself "back" in the 1990s.) The staff I spoke to were proud of the clinic's irregularities in this regard: to them, it was a sign of compassion. Stimulation protocol medicines were "found" for those experiencing financial pressure, and free cycles were often given to women who failed to fall pregnant the first few times. They remembered one woman from Scarborough, who kept on coming back month after month to no avail. Everyone liked her, everyone felt for her— so much so that the daughter of another employee volunteered to donate her eggs. These two women never met, but in her forties, the woman from Scarborough eventually got her baby. Ethical risk was compassionate improvisation—and this substitution, or displacement, radiated out through all areas of the clinic. Laboratory tools (like glass pipettes of a certain diameter for ICSI) weren't commercially available, and so they made their own, melting and shaping glass themselves. Professional accreditation for embryologists didn't really exist. The current head embryologist of Bourn Hall, Adam Burnley, was hired directly from high school; he had passed one A level (biology), and had applied for jobs in a garage and a sugar factory. He learned how to take blood samples by practicing on Mike Macnamee, now the chief executive of the clinic. These were not days of replicability and efficiency, in the way Huxley envisaged, but days of singularity and inefficiency. It was one way to humanize the miracle of outsourcing conception. Nearly everyone I spoke to had worked at Bourn Hall for decades, and spoke with deep feeling for their patients. Their job was righteous; they were helping women become mothers, completing families. They referred to a "natural" need for children, how good it felt to make that dream come true.

Shahzad texted me: Anika was crying, hungry. He was still in the dining room. He had set up his laptop at a table, strapped Anika into the sling, and was bouncing up and down on the giant green exercise ball we had brought with us. This ball was the one thing that would reliably settle Anika, and we had no shame about bringing it everywhere: airports, restaurants, trains, and now, Bourn Hall. They cut a somewhat surprising figure: Shahzad, long and brown in his uniform gray fleece onesie, wearing large headphones, pounding the keyboard, and Anika's tiny hands poking out of either side of the sling, the two of them bouncing so hard you felt sick if you tried to focus on them. I decoupled Anika, and found a wheelchair-accessible toilet to sit in and breastfeed. Anika pulled at my breast, drinking long deep gulps, concentrating, then slowing down, visibly at peace. I could smell the kitchen: they were making some kind of cheese dish for lunch. Back in the dining room, we sat together, eating egg sandwiches, watching the wind in the grass and trees outside. There were obvious signs that much of the initial conservatism that structured the clinic had been put to one side. In 2013, a plaque was added to the building that noted that Jean Purdy was also a co-founder of the clinic. On their website, they now featured stories of same-sex parents and surrogacy. Bourn Hall was also extending itself, partnering with five other clinics in the South East of Britain, and setting up clinics in the United Arab Emirates. But eating in the dining room, listening to the murmur of nurses and doctors and families around me, it still felt like a place to sequester yourself.

THE DAY AFTER Louise Brown was born in 1980, a reporter visited the gynecological surgeon Howard Jones and his wife, Georgeanna

Jones, a reproductive endocrinologist, as they unpacked boxes in the driveway of their new home in Norfolk, Virginia. They had just retired from their positions at John Hopkins University, and Eastern Virginia Medical School had hired them to helm the Department of Obstetrics and Gynecology. Had they heard the news of the world's first IVF baby? Did they think that was possible in the United States? Howard replied, without thinking too much: Yes. All it would take was money. The next day, a check for $5,000 arrived from a former patient who had been treated by Georgeanna; she had read the news report, and wanted to help other women. Within months, they had raised $25,000.

In some ways, the founding of the Joneses' clinic echoed Edwards, Steptoe, and Purdy's: there was the usefulness of private donations, and a division of responsibility between the two directors. The Joneses had the distinct advantage of a preexisting medical school that was far bigger and better equipped than Oldham Hospital. Edwards and Howard Jones had even collaborated in 1965, when Edwards had traveled to the United States and was looking for a more consistent supply of oocytes. In return, the Joneses had visited Cambridge. While Edwards was supportive of their efforts, he was cagey about the exact composition of the culture he was using, as well as other technical specifications. The Joneses were on their own in developing techniques and materials, such as the exact ratio of carbon dioxide, nitrogen, and oxygen that was needed in the incubators to approximate the human body. Every step of the process was subsequently rethought and reconfigured. The Joneses experimented with a shaker unit in the incubator, to mimic the movement of the fallopian tube, in which an egg is continually stirred by tiny hairs (cilia) and by muscular contractions of the tubal wall. They invested in a computer database (with a memory of a whopping 8K), established strict lab procedures, and invented a new aspiration needle. How thin was too thin for a needle to aspirate follicular fluid? Howard Jones decided to try a slightly different laparoscopic technique than Steptoe: rather than inflate the abdomen with nitrogen gas to aid inspection, and make three small abdominal punctures to introduce the laparoscope, Jones decided to use carbon dioxide instead, and make only one puncture with manipulating forceps. Edwards had assumed that IVF would remain an inpatient procedure, but Georgeanna was convinced that gonadotropins could be used, which could increase the number of eggs extracted, as well as standardize the timing of operations. Patients would then have the flexibility to visit the clinic once a day.

For almost a year, they had no luck: in 1980, they removed 19 oocytes from 41 women, 13 of which fertilized, but none progressed to a clinical pregnancy. It wasn't necessarily surprising: it had taken Edwards and Steptoe ten years. In his memoir, *In Vitro Fertilization Comes to America,* Jones characterized this lack of success as having nothing to do with one particular variable, but rather with how finely tuned the lab needed to be in controlling a large number of variables (medium, incubation, sterility procedures, etc.). His account made very visible the fact that a team of embryologists, technicians, anesthetists, and surgeons had to learn to work together. This was happening at Bourn Hall, of course, but Edwards and Steptoe's account essentially ended when Bourn Hall began.

There are many stories told about the beginnings of IVF, but not so many about its middle—and even the ones written by those in the middle tended to emphasize their beginnings. (John Leeton's memoir *Test Tube Revolution: The Early History of IVF*, about the first

IVF pregnancies in Australia, is almost comically focused on his competition with the Joneses and Edwards and Steptoe.) In the rush to document a set of firsts—the first IVF baby born in America, the first born in the Southern Hemisphere, the first set of twins, the first vaginal delivery, the first from a frozen embryo—what was obscured was the rapidly expanding scale of the industry. By the time the Joneses celebrated their first IVF baby, less than a year and a half after Louise Brown, *one hundred women* were already pregnant around the world through IVF, and hoping to carry to term. At least five American clinics were already treating women. Waiting lists at all of these clinics immediately ranged from six months to three years, despite the fact that the success rate then was approximately 5 percent. By 1984, there were clinics operating in France, Austria, Sweden, Italy, Germany, the Netherlands, Switzerland, Australia, Israel, Japan, Yugoslavia, Belgium, Finland, and Canada. In the United States alone, there were sixty-one. Media coverage tended to focus on the stories of patients whose treatment appeared to violate conventional norms: the sixty-two-year-old woman who fell pregnant through IVF, for example, or a woman who used a cousin's egg in place of her own. These stories relied on a brief depth charge of transgression, but the broader interpretive arc remained stubbornly the same: some comment about a slippery slope, another about shifting ethical sands. There was surprisingly little curiosity about the clinics; their structural development, their norms, their expectations for patients were considered a given, just the way it was. The narrative thread of the industry appeared to disappear, like a river into the desert, running out into threads and tributaries, their multiplicity undermining any coherency.

This benefited clinics in the United States, where the anti-abortion lobby was active from the very beginning in trying to block IVF. Groups tried to stop the Joneses' embryology lab from receiving the Certificate of Need it would need to operate, and a public hearing on the matter in 1979 attracted protesters, newspapers, and TV crews, as well as a substantial number of medical students, who arrived very early and filled up the auditorium so that protesters couldn't. *The Virginian-Pilot*, a local newspaper, incorrectly claimed that the clinic would discard defective human embryos, and force women to abort any abnormal fetuses. Georgeanna successfully sued the newspaper for defamation, and was awarded $5.5 million in damages—money that she promptly directed back into the program.

From the 1970s onward, the National Institutes of Health convened a number of panels which included physicians, lawyers, public interest advocates, ethicists, and theologians to discuss new reproductive technologies, but their focus was not so much whether reproductive technologies could continue as much as whether the government should *fund* it. To a non-American, this is a crucial distinction, and one that strikes me as often overlooked in literature on the subject. Private industry has *always* been expected to go its own way in the United States; "national" guidelines that have been debated are not really national as much as applied only to federally funded organizations. As a result, no matter how stringent any commission's finding, the morality it constructed was always incomplete, almost circumvented. Some states outlawed IVF, and others permitted it. Judy Carr, the first woman to give birth to an IVF baby in the United States, would travel from her home state of Massachusetts, where IVF was illegal, to Virginia, where it was allowed.

In the UK, the industry developed differently. In 1982, the British government announced they were appointing a commission to develop guiding principles for the control and regulation of new reproductive technologies. The philosopher Mary Warnock was appointed committee chair, and for the next two years, she worked with obstetricians, gynecologists, scientists, social workers, adoption services, theologians, neurologists, lawyers, and psychiatrists, inviting formal submissions from almost 1,000 organizations and individuals, and receiving 695 public submissions. There was no distinction to be made between public and private medical practice, no natural opt-out clause for parts of the industry. And so the report explicitly tried to articulate a collective point of view on the subject, establishing a range of positions on each issue, carefully describing the grounds for support or disagreement, then offering the inquiry's reasoning. Theirs, Warnock wrote, was a "steady and general point of view," one that tried to "give due consideration both to public and to private morality."

The Warnock Report enshrined, in many ways, a conservative vision of the family. They thought it "better" that a child be raised in a stable relationship between a woman and a man (rather than by a solo parent, or a same-sex couple), though they did not limit parenthood to marriage. (This heteronormative, cisgendered preference was one of the few in the report that was not accompanied by a full reasoning.) The report was particularly worried about "the introduction of a third party into the marriage"—where the insertion of donor eggs or sperm into the body "violates the exclusive physical union of man and wife, and represents a break in the marriage vows." Gamete donation might, the report suggested, be comparable to adultery—though it conceded, noting the precedent of stepparents, that a non–genetically related parent need not be a threat to the stability of the child-parent relationship. Nonetheless, the report insisted that prospective parents *not* know where their donor sperm or eggs came from, nor should donors know who had received their gametes. They disapproved of the (American) notion that couples could "pick" donors based on supplied narratives. They were even more disapproving of surrogacy. Not only did it outsource reproduction in a particularly corporeal way to a third party outside the couple; the report emphasized that payment for such a service would take advantage of economically vulnerable women who had little to sell but their womb. They recommended that surrogacy not be allowed by any licensed agent (for profit or not-for-profit) and that if people pursued this path privately, it should be made law that "all surrogacy agreements are illegal contracts and therefore unenforceable in the courts." In other words, the Warnock Report wanted some things to remain exclusive. A human being's ability to genetically reproduce was a biological assertion of limits, a way to "naturally" construct a morality rooted in the body. What the report did not acknowledge was how it had understood "natural" to mean a stable monogamous relationship between a man and a woman, rather than single or queer parenting.

But the Warnock Report was remarkably scientifically oriented in its definition of human life. It identified one of its tasks as determining an experimental limit for embryos: How old was too old for scientific experimentation? At what point did an embryo become an individual with (depending on your belief structure) a soul? The inquiry noted that a number of developmental milestones might be considered as a limit to experimentation and provided a careful outline of embryonic development. In the very first days of fertilization, when the number of cells in an embryo are few, the cells are totipotent—that is, they can develop into all the different kinds of tissues and organs that make up our bodies, as well as the placenta and fetus. The embryo can even divide in this early stage, and two separate embryos (identical twins) can form. At this point, the embryo is human potential, human clay. It is singular in the sense that it has a singular DNA profile, but it is not a singular being. The embryo is also adrift, moving down the fallopian tube, eventually arriving around day 6 in the uterus, where it begins to implant itself in the uterine wall. This was one limit: at this point, it was understood that even if you managed to cultivate an embryo in a petri dish for longer than 6 days, it would not be able to successfully implant in a human body. At that point, rapid cell division occurs, and the embryo jumps from containing about sixteen cells to between eighty and one hundred. The cell mass looks more differentiated, and you can start to pick out what will become the placenta and fetal membrane. Another limit considered was at 14 or 15 days, when the primitive streak develops; this is the last point at which identical twins can develop from a single embryo. From that point on, cell specialization rapidly increases. By the 17th day, the neural groove appears, which becomes neural folds and then the neural tube. Another limit posed was the beginning of a central nervous system (around 22 or 23 days), which could conceivably be when the embryo might first feel pain (though it is far more likely an embryo would not feel pain until much later, when the nervous system actually starts to function). Considering all of these, the Warnock Report finally settled on 14 days as the cutoff point, just before the appearance of the primitive streak "marks the beginning of individual development of the embryo." Even at this point, a woman could miscarry and not think it was anything other than her normal menstrual cycle. (Indeed, this is the reason it's hard to accurately establish what percentage of pregnancies end in miscarriages.)

The Warnock Report recommended the formation of a licensing body to which scientists, IVF clinics, and research labs could apply for approval. All procedures carried out in any clinic in the United Kingdom would be recorded. Further, the report insisted that the licensing body be composed of both scientists and "lay person[s]." In doing so, they established basic assumptions about the transparency of best practice and the necessity of multiple points of view as a public health responsibility. These were not easy decisions to make: the committee was so divided that three appendices of dissenting opinions were attached to the report (one for surrogacy, one against all experimentation on embryos, and one against the creation of embryos for research purposes). But these dissenting opinions gave greater weight to the committee's findings: the center appeared to hold precisely because dissent *was* registered, and knew its place. In her foreword to the report, Warnock noted that although there were differences of opinion, everyone also noted that their minds had changed as they progressed through the material. This seemed a crucial point to her: everyone had experienced both fluidity and fixity in their thinking, and everyone had expected to both change their mind and not give up on the need for principle. She observed that in general, people wished for some sense of containment, no matter what: "the very existence of morality depends on it. A society which has no inhibiting limits, especially in the areas with which we have been concerned, questions of birth and death, of the setting up of families, and the valuing of human life, would be a society without moral scruples. *And this nobody wants* [emphasis hers]." The anthropologist Marilyn Strathern has termed the United Kingdom's collective agreement on developmental markers and definitions a "cultural education": the public might not have known these details of embryonic development before the report was released, but the media certainly publicized them, and established a set of propositions that could be debated.

In the United States, there has been no such governmentally directed "cultural education," though there were, from the 1970s on, a series of commissions that recommended embryonic research be allowed to proceed, and that even settled on the same 14-day limit. They did this knowing that any actual application to carry out federally funded in vitro embryonic development would be stymied by a maze of regulatory practices. Their vacillation was also driven by debates about gene splicing in the 1970s and stem-cell research in the 1980s. Both seemed to be technologies with huge potential—and great risk. Scientists initiated their own research moratorium on gene splicing in 1974 (worried about the ability to weaponize illness). Though a moratorium was never suggested for stem-cell research, the cost was obvious: a line of stem cells (which were pluripotent, and could become *anything*—brain cells, blood cells, bone marrow cells, muscle cells, all in all, replacement tissue) necessitated the killing of the embryo. Not all embryos produced viable stem-cell lines, either; you would have to kill many to develop a few.

In the early 1990s, it appeared that there was a chance to more publicly define what an embryo was (and define its rights) with the election of Bill Clinton, the first Democratic president since 1981. Two years into his tenure, President Clinton convened a Human Embryo Research Panel to comprehensively review the government's position on a number of areas in embryology, including stem-cell research. A number of Republican politicians were even swayed enough by the promise of stem-cell research that they advocated *for* it to the panel. Yet this report ended up being just as ineffectual as the others had been: Clinton, beset by other moral quandaries of his own making, lost momentum and political goodwill. He decided that advancing stem-cell research just wasn't worth the headache, anticipating, in part, the pro-life lobby, and his own administration refused to back the report's findings. Clinton thereby alienated a large number of research scientists who concluded they would never be able to do their research in federally funded institutions regardless of which party held the White House, Senate, and Congress. They had already been moving into the arms of unregulated private industry, and now it became the sensible choice for young researchers who weren't particularly interested in a career in academia. Another consequence was that there have been far fewer American scientists actively involved in establishing and extending a public debate about reproductive technologies. In the United States, broad definitions of scientific and public health authority—of who gets to decide—were ceded to the stridency of pro-life and pro-choice movements, who figured reproductive ethics as a zero-sum game, with no fluidity to their thinking.

At the same time, the IVF industry was flourishing, checked only by a self-imposed sense of ethical restraint. Professional societies like the Society for Assisted Reproductive Technology (SART) and the American Society for Reproductive Medicine (ASRM) began to collaborate in setting lab standards. In 1992, they helped to implement the Fertility Clinic Success Rate and Certification Act of 1992, which required all clinics to submit an annual report to the Centers for Disease Control. But the CDC had no legal wherewithal to check the accuracy of this information: it was data collection without teeth. This is one of the main reasons why we don't know how many IVF babies have been born in the United States. There was (and is) no legal restriction on the type of research that could be done privately: if you wanted to create 5-day-old embryos specifically for research purposes, using gametes from donors, you could. It was only the biological limits of implantation—the fact that embryos need the uterine environment to grow beyond 13 days—that might stop you.

It was not surprising that commercial expansion resulted in ethical risk. There were cases of embryos being stolen or given to the wrong people. Less extreme, but far more pervasive, was the practice of implanting multiple embryos at once, increasing the chances of pregnancy, but also the chance of multiple births and with it, the chance of maternal and fetal health complications. Between 1980 and 2000, the rate of twins rose 300 percent and triplets by 700 percent. The nuclear family compressed itself into an ever denser spacing of time and children. A family of multiples could be achieved with one pregnancy. This was deeply appealing to patients who had been trying for years, had little time "left," and were desperate to avoid yet another cycle. If you have three embryos that will not live past three days, what would you do? For much of the 1990s there was no reliable way to tell which embryos would successfully implant and which wouldn't, though some clinics engaged in visually "grading" embryos in terms of cellular shape. (The ability to gauge embryo potential today is still a contested subject.) It was, by all accounts, an inexact science. Most patients, focused intently only on falling pregnant, considered multiple births an acceptable risk to simply achieve a pregnancy. Clinics acknowledged there were health risks to multiple births, but did not elaborate. Obstetricians complained that they were left to deal with the results of IVF's willful optimism.

In her book *Everything Conceivable*, Liza Mundy documented numerous stories of health complications during the pregnancy and birth of multiples. It is one thing to hear abstract statistics, and another to confront the actual outcomes for women who lose a child, or who realize that their child will never be independent, no matter how old they grow. Mundy described, for example, a family who did not leave the house for the first year of their quadruplets' lives unless it was to visit the doctor: life beyond basic health needs was just too complicated to organize. Given these risks, some embryologists' stories about the 1990s appear almost criminal. Lucinda Veeck Gosden recalled one practice transferring 17 embryos into one woman. Mark Evans, who still practices selective reduction in multiples—the injection of potassium chloride into the hearts of one or more fetuses in utero—recalled seeing the ultrasound of a woman pregnant with 12 fetuses. (Her doctor had only told her about 6.) These may be extreme outliers, but in the 1980s and 1990s it was routine to implant between 4 and 6 embryos.

OTHER COUNTRIES MOVED in very different legislative directions from the United States. In Belgium, for instance, there are legal limits on how many embryos can be implanted; if you are younger than thirty-six years old, for example, you *cannot* implant more than one embryo for your first and second cycle. This restriction—and the hospital savings from the reduction in multiple births—actually funds the guarantee of *six* free cycles of IVF for every Belgian woman younger than forty-eight who cannot conceive. These parameters help recast the economic privilege of IVF: it is not individual, but national, a right of citizenship.

One of the doctors who helped draft an early iteration of this legislation was Willem Ombelet, a South African gynecologist who moved in 1987 to Genk, a small town to the northeast of Brussels, to begin an IVF clinic in the hospital there. The contrast must've been striking. For years, he had worked in townships in Pretoria offering mobile medical services and had seen both ends of the fertility spectrum there: some women pulled him aside, desperate to conceive, and others wanted to put an end to their fertility. For both groups, it was a hushed conversation; children are seen, unequivocally, as a blessing, and the lack of them as a sign of punishment by the gods. In Africa, the percentage of women who identify with the statement that "the ideal number of children is zero" has *always* been less than 2 percent. Cultural traditions are often predicated on children; in Nigeria and Cameroon, land claims are negotiated through the number of children. In Nigeria, women lose their right to inherit their husband's property if there are no children. Women are nearly always held responsible for the lack of children in a marriage, despite the fact that 50 percent of all infertility is quite possibly male-factor.

In 2001, at a WHO meeting, two researchers proposed a continuum of social suffering to measure the effects of infertility. The language is banal, but the extraordinary pathos remains. In the developed world, couples tend to experience social suffering in level 1 (fear, guilt, self-blame) through level 2 (marital stress, depression, helplessness) and level 3 (mild marital or social violence and abuse, social alienation)—but in the developing world, this extends to level 4 (severe economic deprivation, moderate to severe violence, total loss of social status), level 5 (violence-induced suicide, starvation/

disease), and level 6 (lost dignity in death). Women face complete economic, social, and physical isolation. They are routinely abandoned if they cannot give birth. There is a region in Egypt where you literally lose your name if you cannot fall pregnant. Women like myself, in America, have the privilege of keeping their grief private. It is a humbling readjustment to realize just how much further your grief and pain could extend.

The rate of infertility worldwide seems to hover at approximately 10 percent, but its causes change according to where you live. This percentage might also increase because of cases of secondary infertility—that is, women who can conceive a first child, but not a second. In many countries in sub-Saharan Africa, more than 30 percent of women experience secondary infertility, the consequence of infection from postpartum trauma, sexually transmitted diseases, and abortion. Reproductive health in the region is generally very poor: overall, from 65 percent to 85 percent of women in the sub-Saharan region suffer from some form of tubal block, which might range from polycystic fibrosis to poor uterine health. The rate tends to be only anecdotally established because of the social stigma attached to diagnosis. Nonetheless, a 2004 study by the World Health Organization estimated that in the developing world, 186 million women suffered from infertility.

Upon moving to Genk, Ombelet found it hard to forget that Belgium's state-supported infertility care is at least indirectly possible because of Belgium's colonial rule of the Congo from the late nineteenth century to the early 1960s. Much of the wealth from rubber and ivory, acquired at gunpoint and machete tip, was spent on numerous programs of public building in Brussels, Ostend, and Antwerp—precisely the buildings that Ombelet passed by every day on his way to Genk Hospital. In general, the extensive social services offered by Belgium were only possible because of the deaths of millions half a world and more than a century away. Despite the UN Universal Declaration of Human Rights, which states that "Men and women of full age . . . have the right to marry and to found a family," IVF is mostly considered a privilege for the wealthy, the well-insured, or those living in a country with a generous social safety net. The geographical concentration of that wealth is striking. Europe and the United Kingdom account for 35 percent of IVF births in the world. The United States, Mexico, and Canada account for another 27 percent. Africa—the *continent*—accounts for 0.5 percent of IVF births. There has always been some variation in the price; in the US, the average cost is around $12,000 per cycle, and in the Czech Republic, $3,000—which has created a burgeoning industry in IVF tourism as the middle class from one country take advantage of another's—but this sliding scale is still out of reach for all but the singularly rich in Africa. These inequities are stark: in the Republic of Congo, the average life span is almost thirty years less than it is in Belgium, infant mortality is 24 times higher, and infertility affects almost double the women there. Though the Congo's birth rate is 3 times higher than Belgium's, the physical and emotional costs of birth—infant death, secondary infertility, and other physical complications—remain extraordinarily high.

These kinds of discrepancies motivated Ombelet. In 2007, he convened a three-day conference about infertility in the developing world in Arusha, a city in Tanzania, chosen because of its proximity to the Olduvai Gorge, where the oldest human remains have been discovered. Nearly two hundred people from NGOs, universities, newspapers, hospitals, and infertility clinics met to register and document the problem of infertility and to consider ways to address it. By the end, everyone agreed there were three possible routes. The first was to develop a one-day clinic that could diagnose common causes of infertility by conducting basic blood work—to measure hormone levels and detect hepatitis B and C and tuberculosis—and cervical smears, hysterosalpingography, vaginal ultrasounds, and/or mini-hysteroscopy (to examine the uterine lining). Within a day, a woman could understand why she wasn't falling pregnant. Some of these issues are relatively easily addressed using medication; others require surgery. But women, at the very least, would understand the scale of infertility they were facing. For men, along with blood tests, a fresh sample of semen could be washed and evaluated for count and motility. The second option was to make widely available fertility drugs that would mildly stimulate the ovaries. The third option was to open IVF centers.

It was as they explored the third option that, a year later, Ombelet and Dr. Sheryl van der Poel from the World Health Organization contacted Professor Jonathan Van Blerkom, an embryologist and professor at the University of Colorado Boulder. They were on the hunt for hand-me-down IVF equipment and thought he might help. Van Blerkom was skeptical; even if they were to find such equipment, it wouldn't be easy to maintain in countries where power surges and outages were common. But months later, he was struck by an idle thought while driving home. As a graduate student in the 1970s, his job had been driving rabbit and pig embryos from Arizona to Colorado. They were kept alive in a very simple combination of sodium bicarbonate, water, and citric acid. It was relatively easy to monitor the pH balance; if it got too high, he just needed to inject some CO_2. You could, he reasoned, do the same with human embryos. He also had a thought about how you might generate that CO_2. As a child, one of his favorite toys was a plastic scuba diver he'd purchased with box tops from Kellogg's Corn Flakes. One chamber of the tank was filled with vinegar, and the other with baking soda. As the contents reacted with each other, they gave off CO_2, causing the diver to dip and resurface, releasing bubbles. Van Blerkom wondered if you could keep an embryo alive using the same technique.

The chemistry seemed ludicrously simple. In a conventional IVF clinic, approximately 35 percent of running costs are spent in the laboratory. Some of this is diagnostic blood and semen work, but then there are the considerable operating costs of an embryo lab, which include staffing, equipment, and maintenance. Incubators are extremely costly, as are air purifiers and ventilation hoods. But Ombelet and Van Blerkom rethought a few basic assumptions. What would happen if you reduced the number of times an embryo was moved from one receptacle to another, or removed from the incubator for observation? You wouldn't need quite the same emphasis on air quality control, and you wouldn't need as many trained embryologists. They reasoned that it was quite possible to combine sperm and egg in the test tube, and leave the ensuing embryo to grow rather than removing the excess sperm. They also thought it quite possible to find a microscope that would work well enough through glass. If this was true, then the only remaining requirement was a consistent temperature, and this was relatively easy to achieve with a minimum of equipment.

The result was an embryology kit that fits inside a shoebox and that looked, with its modest metal casing, glass tubing, and basic cork stoppers, a lot like a high school science experiment. The materials barely cost more than $10. It was then a matter of establishing whether such a low-cost method worked as well as conventional IVF. In order to persuade the Belgian Ethics Committee, Ombelet designed a study wherein couples under age thirty-six and with a sperm count of more than a million received ovarian stimulation. If the oocytes harvested numbered more than eight, half were fertilized and cultured the usual way, and the other half using the new method. An independent embryologist, blinded as to which were which, would then select the best embryos to implant, and the others would be frozen. The results were remarkable. Using conventional IVF resulted in a 29 percent live birth rate. Using this new method, it was 30.4 percent. Sixteen live births resulted from embryos that had been cultured using this low-cost method.

The implications for the developing world were clear. If you could find a clinician to prescribe a hormone stimulation protocol, who was also able to carry out laparoscopic surgery, you could conduct IVF anywhere. IVF could cost less than 500 euros. André Van Steirteghem, one of the key figures in the development of ICSI (the injection of sperm directly into an ovum), called it the third revolution in IVF. When Ombelet's team published their results in 2012, they rightly assumed a flurry of media interest, and with it, the prospect of increased funding and the chance to roll out low-cost IVF centers throughout the developing world. Yet though the trials were widely reported on in the press, the money never came. Then came additional bureaucratic hurdles that were almost laughable in their banality. The test tubes, stoppers, and medium they were using were not CE accredited in the EU (which is equivalent to being FDA approved). They had to redo their trial with new materials. It took years to replicate the same results.

The knee-jerk reaction of many people in the developed world to the prospect of infertility care in the developing world seems to be mild outrage; the world is already overburdened as it is, and we hardly need more children we cannot feed. On a list of health priorities in these countries (HIV prevention, malaria, clean water), infertility seems less consequential. Yet maybe, if you conceive of infertility care as part of a broader program of reproductive health, you can start to sense its importance. If you want women to make mindful decisions about how many children to have (and when to have them), they need to know that they can be medically supported should they choose to delay pregnancy. They need to be able to diagnose the cause of their infertility, to understand if it is the result of a treatable infection, or male-factor infertility. It should not have to remain a mystery. To assume that women in the developing world cannot be trusted with this kind of information—that they will simply use IVF to unthinkingly give birth to more and more children—is to resort to a caricature of female passivity and stoicism that has more to do with a neocolonial condescension than anything else.

I visited Willem Ombelet in 2016, days after I had visited Bourn Hall: Shahzad, Anika, and I caught a high-speed train from London to Brussels, bouncing in the aisle on our giant green ball. Two years earlier, Ombelet had begun a partnership with the Pentecostal Church in Ghana, which had built an IVF clinic. Ghanaian doctors and technicians were recruited and flown to Genk for training. There had been two "missions," when Ombelet and his team had flown to Ghana and worked alongside their Ghanaian counterparts trying to recreate the success of the Belgian trials. But there had been minimal success. In the first trial, they underestimated the number of women who were suffering from uterine polyps and myoma (fibroids) that blocked the implantation of an embryo. In a Belgian population, this condition would be relatively rare, but in Ghana, more than 70 percent of women had some form of uterine scarring regardless of their age, and Ombelet and his team did not think to give them all a hysteroscopy prior to treatment. They also used limited air filtration. In the second mission, they discovered that the doctor who had been seeing the women prior to their cycle, and who had prescribed the pill to regulate their hormone levels, did not realize the last week's worth of pills were inactive pills designed to bring on a woman's menstrual cycle. The women had started their stimulation protocol a week later in their cycle than they should have, so their uterine lining wasn't thick enough when it came time for the embryos to implant.

These complications were depressingly simple: Ghana needed clinicians who were more experienced in prescribing hormone protocols, and they needed more diagnostic work done on the patients. In other words, they needed a higher standard of preexisting and ongoing patient care. It wasn't enough to only focus on the weeks of stimulation. Ombelet realized that even if low-cost IVF were possible, if it wasn't applied with a certain degree of precision, the success rate would be so low that women would be dissuaded from embarking on a course of treatment. He had overestimated his ability to oversee the process, as well as unthinkingly relied upon a certain standard of care offered by Belgium's medical system.

His subsequent decision seemed, on first glance, to be inimical to the initial impulse of his project. Ombelet *did* have to create a set of air quality and microscope controls—and he insisted that, going forward, any center interested in using his technique must also install this equipment. The result was to lower the setup costs from

1.5 million–3 million euros to 300,000–500,000 euros; a sizable drop, but still hardly a small cost. The overall issue had become one of replicable infrastructure rather than design. He told me that he had received expressions of interest from China, India, and Colombia—but that everyone was waiting to see what might happen in Ghana.

The day I visited, he had received bad news: an IVF pregnancy in Ghana had ended in miscarriage. At lunchtime, I watched him give a presentation to his colleagues. Ten or so nurses and doctors sat around the table in the staff room, unwrapping their sandwiches, watching Ombelet as he ran through his PowerPoint, listing key statistics, describing his treatment protocol and study results, insisting on the importance of funding. His audience seemed detached. They listened politely and ate their food, checking their phones discreetly. There were no questions at the end. I asked a nurse afterward how she felt about it. "Dr. Ombelet has been giving the same presentation for years now. And it is always 'Next year, next year,'" she said. "He has been waiting for a birth, for it all to happen. And it hasn't." Ombelet had the air of a man waiting for a train that should have come a long time ago. Still he waited, peering anxiously into the distance, reluctant to leave his spot, quietly furious that the universe had not yet provided. He spoke of plans to roll out low-cost IVF in London and Portugal by the end of this year, essentially offering it as a cheaper option at already-established IVF clinics: maybe the road to addressing infertility in Africa would be paved by the working class in the developed world. But he knew that this would also meet resistance: Why would the IVF industry want their patients to opt for a $2,000 treatment when they would pay $12,000 USD?

It's true that a lower price point would increase patient numbers, but Ombelet's approach to IVF also challenges a number of basic tenets held by standard IVF clinics. Right now, many clinics favor high-stimulation protocols, essentially prescribing large doses of hormones to stimulate egg production. His version of low-cost IVF assumed it is better to stress the body as little as possible, with minimal stimulation, which lowers the number of eggs harvested. Clinics also assume a certain threshold amount of sperm cells are needed for each fertilization attempt (at least 1 million spermatozoa per ml of seminal fluid, of which at least 30 percent are motile, 15 percent have progressive motility, and 20 have normal morphology), whereas low-cost IVF argues that successful fertilization can be achieved with a sperm count as low as 10,000 motile sperm cells. Standard clinics argue that the remaining sperm cannot be left with a fertilized egg for days on end; Ombelet's studies suggest otherwise. Low-cost IVF poses a number of challenges to conventional thinking, and complicates the path to pregnancy by offering yet another option that patients will have to consider as part of their treatment plan. The net result would be a view of IVF as a series of successively aggressive options rather than the current go-for-broke mentality that many women are encouraged to cultivate, myself included.

I asked Ombelet how much money he actually needed to establish a few working clinics in the developing world, with trained clinicians and appropriate equipment. His answer was laughably low for the systemic change it offered: less than $10 million USD. He had approached a number of different organizations for funding, and though there was polite interest, no funding had materialized. The number of private IVF clinics in Ghana and across Africa continues to rise, and though their treatment costs are lower than in the developed world, they are still only financially accessible to the top 2 percent of earners. Ombelet's technology would make IVF accessible to the African middle class, and though this would appear to be an untapped, lucrative market, it is not in the IVF industry's broader interests to make room for a process that would substantially upend their own cost and profit calculations.

Ombelet has tried to make the gains visible, commissioning mini-documentaries of low-cost IVF in Ghana. There are shots of the Pentecost Hospital at Madina being built, brick by brick; shots of Accra, dust, tangled rebar, children tied onto their mothers' backs, open air clinics where women wait, fanning themselves. There is footage of Ghanaian clinicians in winter coats, walking up the steps of the Sint-Jan Hospital in Genk, Belgium, ready to be trained. We see the same clinicians back in Ghana, examining the eggs and sperm from each couple. Bourn Hall and the Pentecost Hospital at Madina could not look more different from each other, and are striking representations of the economic privilege that Edwards and Steptoe quietly relied on, and Ombelet cannot. Remember: all the Joneses had to do was tell a reporter that starting a clinic would just take money, and a check arrived the next day in the mail. The visual reality of Ombelet's attempt to reverse the colonial legacy of centuries of medical and economic privilege is quietly remarkable. Over and over again, Ombelet tells the camera that the Walking Egg project is named for an egg that doesn't know borders, that enjoys universal global access to fertility care. Dr. Nathalie Dhont, who has worked across Africa as a gynecologist focusing on reproductive health and infertility, mildly reminds the camera: "It's not what we think is important, but what they [Ghanaian women] think is important."

Before he drove me back to the train station, Ombelet wanted to show me something else, he said—the work of an old friend, a conceptual artist. We turned off the main road and headed toward his studio. This friend, Koen Vanmechelen, a Belgian, had been working on eggs for decades too. Vanmechelen and Ombelet had first met in 1993, at an andrology conference. They hit it off: both men fervently believed in the power of art to inform science, and vice versa. In 2000, they began publishing the magazine *The Walking Egg*, which was distributed to infertility specialists worldwide. I was intrigued: How could I not be? It was one of the first times, in my research, that I had seen the frank acknowledgment that two very different discourses *could* speak to one another directly and learn from each other.

Vanmechelen's studio turned out also to be a gallery, and it was also called the Open University of Diversity, housed in a beautifully restored nineteenth-century gelatin factory in Genk. Our shoes clacked on the poured concrete floor. One of his most long-standing projects (begun in 1997) was the Cosmopolitan Chicken Project, which involved crossbreeding national chicken breeds that had long been kept apart, deliberately creating hybrids which he then photographed. There were perhaps 40 portraits of these chickens in the studio (though more than 3,000 had been taken by then). Their eyes had the candor and regard of any fine portrait, their gaze beseeching in a way that I suspect neither they nor we could entirely understand. Here were other walking eggs, but it all felt so literal. It pained me that Vanmechelen had obviously raised millions of dollars to crossbreed chickens for a conceptual art project, while Ombelet could not do the same for African women suffering from infertility. The world's priorities felt ghastly.

The chickens were barely the beginning: scattered throughout the rooms were various stuffed and sculpted vivisectionist fantasies. Here was a peacock with the skull of a cow. There was a Medusa's head, where the woman's face was clearly African, and the snakes' heads had been replaced by chickens'. I struggled to know what to do with my face. How could Ombelet, who had dedicated decades of his life to addressing disparities of reproductive health care between the North and South, *not* see the overtones of Vanmechelen's work? In one giant photo on one wall, Vanmechelen, bare-chested, wearing a full-length coat made of chicken heads, stood in the desert, holding the reins of a dun-colored camel. He was gazing longingly at a woman of African descent on the other side of the composition, sitting on green grass and holding a white camel. The two images had been spliced together: one taken in the United Arab Emirates, the other in Belgium. It was his photo editing that had created the romance; she hadn't been looking at him until he retroactively made it so. He may have thought it was an inverted interracial romance (he was South, she was North), but you could still feel the unthinking force of his hand, his assumption that this look between them would be just as charged for the viewer as it was to him. His work was a painfully contemporary representation of centuries of colonial thinking. I told myself that I was wrong, that I was rushing to judgment. Ombelet had been so kind, giving me most of his day, taking the time to talk to me when, half a world away, a woman was mourning the possibility of a child that was alive, and then was not. Shahzad was texting me. Anika was hungry. I caught the train back, breasts aching with milk, watching the buildings flash past, newly uneasy about my own desire to write about anyone else's roving fertility.

A week later, Shahzad, Anika, and I were in the Czech Republic: Shahzad was recording an album with an old friend in a studio two hours' drive from Prague. During the day I'd bounce on the green ball, writing up the notes of my trip, or walk in the forests and rural roads around the studio. I couldn't stop anxiously thinking about Vanmechelen's art. Here was a self-proclaimed union of subjective art and objective science, and it enthusiastically echoed the economic and racial privilege at the heart of Western scientific exploration. And how different was I, really? I was also reframing ethical risk as compassionate improvisation. Always, Anika was strapped to me, her little face lying against my breastbone. When I had chosen to undergo IVF, I had focused on it as a technology rather than an industry, and preferred to understand my risks as private rather than public. I had directly benefited from the risks the industry had taken, and here I was, a white woman wandering along empty roads with my child. I look at the photos I took of those days, and think about Vanmechelen's poses as well as my own. Here was my sleeping child's face: here was mine. As a feminist, my own ease of movement as a woman means so much to me, but this is a freedom oiled by privilege. Weeks later, I spoke with Vanmechelen on the phone; he had heard of my visit, and was perfectly happy to be interviewed. We spoke mostly of the 2016 presidential election. He was content to offer sound bites: I, in turn, was content to note them down, and never directly challenge him. He was standing too close to my own fault lines.

Eleven months later, in September 2017, a baby boy was born in Ghana, the result of Ombelet's low-cost IVF methods. It was the third attempt for the couple, who had been infertile for eight years. Ombelet has done it: he and his team have prevailed, dealing with accreditation complications, import duties on equipment, and resistance from the larger IVF industry. The photos of the birth—the baby, surrounded by the all-African medical team, dressed in scrubs—are quietly remarkable, but the press coverage outside of Belgium and Africa has been minimal. Other births have followed since. The door has been opened to reimagining the cost structure of IVF, basic treatment protocols, and who might benefit, and Ombelet continues: commuting to his clinic in Genk, collaborating with his peers in Ghana, presenting his case to anyone who will listen. He has proof of concept now, but remarkably, it seems, people are still waiting.

In the years since, Vanmechelen has built a 22 million–euro ecological park in public-private partnership with the city of Genk. "Labiomista" is essentially a zoo that thinks of itself as an ark: it foregrounds the interplay between domesticity and wildness with "zones" for animals of varying dispositions toward humans. When I visited his studio, they were discussing the future placement of the wolves. The project's attempt to offer a paradigm shift is fueled by Vanmechelen's "transdisciplinary" inclinations. It is a useful attempt to complicate the binary between artificial and natural: this, it seems, is also what a "cultural education" might look like. And yet I still find myself shrinking from it, perhaps because it is so quick to assert its utopian bona fides. I distrust the relief that comes from thinking one has found a solution.

11

LOOK! LOOK!

Before Anika was born, my mind was like a submarine. I would never have put it that way then, but in an eight-hour stretch of working, my brain would slowly descend into a problem or thought, and hours would go by as I slowly worked through it. I would ascend again, look out the window, have a shower, exercise, still thinking, now watching the world, tendrils of the thought still moving through me.

After she was born, my mind felt like one of the squirrels in the backyard; even when I had four hours, I had to dart from one thing to another, never stopping, never staying. The ideas I developed had a different shape to them: a different radius, verticality, depth. There was no way to separate the time of writing from the time of motherhood. I kept on writing, though I sometimes fell asleep sitting upright in the café. I kept on writing, but one hour out of three would be spent frantically buying what we needed online, or filling out yet another form that came with the bureaucracy of birth and buying a home. I kept on writing but I noticed I had stopped reading almost entirely. I kept on writing, but the dishes needed to be done, as well as the laundry and the vacuuming. It was virtually impossible to do a lot of this when she was awake, because she wanted to be held, and would cry if she wasn't, and the one thing that reliably undid me, that turned me into a wreck, was Anika's crying. I kept writing, but she cried a lot.

For the first few months, I slept for three hours at a stretch; eight hours of sleep might be cobbled out of fifteen. I often slept upright, cradling Anika. I knew that this was dangerous behavior, but I had an animal alertness I had never experienced before. My senses were sharpened. I heard the stairs, the door, even the fridge in the kitchen when it cycled on and off. I didn't dream.

Small actions would whip me into a fever of anxious rage. If you have a baby and are out alone in public, and need to pee, there is nowhere to put her; you have to balance her on your knees as you sit on the toilet. If your baby is crying for milk, and you are sitting on a subway, you have a choice: either breastfeed her in front of twenty strangers, at least five of whom will stare at you, or refuse your daughter, and listen to her scream all the way to your destination, watching the backs of people stiffen. I moved apartments with Anika strapped to me, directing the loading and unloading of the contents of my life like an air traffic controller. My maternity leave was going to finish soon, and the only way I could get her to sleep for longer at night was to give her formula or pureed food. It worked, and the intense guilt and joy I felt when I could get her to sleep for five hours without relying on my body was almost as powerful as the night, when she was five months old, when I went on a date, desperate to sit at a bar and have a glass of wine with someone who didn't see me as a mother, who wanted to talk about the world as I had known it before.

This is what James Hillman, whose thoughts on archetypal

psychology found surprising footholds throughout American popular culture in the 1990s, had to say about motherhood, language,
and the imagination:

> As child is equivalent with imagination, the mother's lan-
> guage becomes unimaginative, imperative, abstract. As
> the child is growth, she becomes static and empty, unable
> to react with spontaneous novelty. As the child is time-
> less, eternal, she becomes time-bound, scheduled, hur-
> ried. Her morality becomes one-sidedly responsible and
> disciplinarian. Her sense of future and hope is displaced
> on her actual child; thereby postpartum depression may
> become a chronic undertone. As her actual child carries
> her feelings of vulnerability, she may over-attend to it to
> the neglect of herself, with consequent resentments. Also,
> her thought processes become restricted to adult forms of
> reason so that the ghost voices and faces, animals, the
> scenes of eidetic imagination become estranged and feel
> like pathological delusions and hallucinations. And her
> language loses its emotional and incantational power; she
> explains and argues.

Oh, the certainty. Hillman's right in the sense that it is hard *not* to
undergo an almost chemical, compositional change, but he is wrong
about pretty much everything else.

When Anika was barely two or three weeks old, I bought her
first book for her. It was called *Look Look!* and it included eight black-
and-white graphic illustrations of the following: two hands, the sun,
two faces, two flowers, a car, a cat, a school of fish, stars, and the

moon. I sat with her propped up in my lap, and showed her the pictures, saying the names, quietly marveling that these were the names and objects that a number of people considered crucial. It was, I thought, direct training in some kind of eidetic archetypal. Sources of light. The nonhuman. The human. We read this book hundreds of times: hands, sun, faces, flowers, car, cat, fish, stars, moon; and again; and again. Hillman underestimated how much a mother does *with* an infant rather than just *for* it. When you are teaching your infant to look, you are looking also. With Anika, I relearned the world. Time poured like sand out of all the things I needed to do, and into the experiences she needed. Hours with her felt endless.

As she grew, Anika started to understand the symbolic order: these pictures were of objects that existed in the world. They also had sounds attached to them. At first, she learned animals by the noises they made. The horse went "neeeiiiiggghhhh." The dog went "ruf ruf." (Her Russian friend said "guv guv," because that is how a dog barks in Russian storybooks.) The sheep went "baaaa." Then she began to make the words her own. A whale was not a whale but a "waay-ull." A snake was a "nake." A fish was "psssh." A butterfly was "Biii." She was remarkably precise with some multisyllabic words. "Purple" and "turtle" were said with evident satisfaction. She began to identify objects with pleasure, unprompted. She was particularly fond of spotting the moon, even in the late afternoon. The book's author, Peter Linenthal, was right: Anika adored the smiling face of a sun, suddenly appearing on a shop's awning, or on a tile in a strange kitchen. She found stars on T-shirts and bike helmets. Any walk involved multiple stops to tear a few choice flowers apart.

My own mother Skyped with Anika most weeks, sometimes for

hours, watching my daughter play with her toys in a living room halfway around the world. She had a box of my old toys back in New Zealand, and held them up to the screen, one after another. "What is this, Anika?" she'd ask over and over again, taking obvious pleasure in Anika's ability to name the object across space. She held up an animatronic puppy dog that panted when you pushed its paw, and eight thousand miles away, Anika panted back happily in return.

Though giving birth to Anika moved me beyond the horizon line of my life, it did so in the same way that a cork, rather than corkscrewed out of a bottle, is pushed *inside* it, and now I was confronted by even more basic forms of repetition, which became the most fundamental verbs in my life. Feeding, cleaning, tidying, playing, buying, reading, preparing, feeding, sleeping, wiping, arranging, playing, ordering, reading, feeding. The repetition became ritualistic. With each repeated sentence or action for Anika, I could almost see the neural grooves deepening; it gave her a cognitive steadiness, the faith that some things could be relied upon so she could risk others. Hands, sun, faces, flowers, car, cat, fish, stars, moon. These repetitions could be absurdly mundane. As an adult, I had forsworn curtains (so that I wouldn't have to open and close them), but I found myself purchasing curtains for Anika's bedroom without thinking, and religiously opening and closing them every day. She had a particular bottle, and a particular time for drinking it. She had books just before bed and just after bed. Anika's language and desire began shaping itself around these repetitions; she learned to name them, to demand them, and finally, to relish them, to sigh happily and cuddle me close when they happened. The mundane grew in depth, like a muddy puddle that secretly extended farther down than you expected, into the earth.

By the time she was three, ritual was a way that Anika drew the world close to her, pulling it tight to conform to her shape. She had a particular way of stroking her favorite stuffed animal, Sheepie. She'd cup him loosely in her hand, and thumb his tail, exactly the way someone would finger a set of prayer beads. This would go on for ten minutes at a time and often just before she fell asleep. I lay next to her, marveling at deftly precise movements of her hand. She still couldn't drink something without spilling it, but her hands on Sheepie were miraculously precise. We bought two other copies of the same toy for fear she'd lose Sheepie, but it was already irreplaceable: the original Sheepie was stroked so much it halved in size, compressed or whittled by time and love. With Anika, I was learning the world of objects again, learning to categorize them, aestheticize them, and take solace in them. I started to understand how ritual can be recharged, and how wrong Hillman was; my eidetic imagination had never been closer to me.

IN MY CHILDHOOD home back in New Zealand, there was a large exposed stone chimney that backed onto the kitchen. If you walked around it, into the living room, the fireplace looked naturally impressive—modernly ancient in a 1970s kind of way—but in the kitchen, where everything was Formica and tile, the chimney was a strange addition, stuck between the bench and cupboards, a thing you didn't expect. The rocks were ugly—oddly shaped, jagged, black, and dumpy—but someone had thought well enough of them to make them the feature of the house.

As a child, I would stand in the kitchen with my back against this chimney, watching my father make dinner. He would take a frozen chicken from the freezer and peel off its plastic bag, slipping it into a Perspex glass container with a solid thunk; pry the frozen bird's legs apart and remove the gizzards in their plastic bag, dust the chicken with salt and oil, find the lid, and place the whole thing in the microwave. He'd put water on to boil for the rice, chop the cabbage to steam it. As he cooked, he sang songs from his own childhood, and the cats would watch from the bench, eying the thawing gizzards in the sink. Chicken, cabbage, rice: this is what we ate for dinner most nights.

When the chicken was carved and the cabbage served, I would watch my mother hesitate at the kitchen counter while everyone else sat down at the table to eat. She had just arrived home from work. The light was soft and yellow and strong on her face. She would stand there, while we waited, picking at the chicken carcass with her fingers, plucking at the threads of meat tucked away along the ribs. I recognized then how much she loved to do this, almost without knowing it: how it was the best part of the meal, for me and for her.

My mother's solution to most sicknesses was antibiotics. For a while, she gave me a foul-tasting antibiotic called Augmentin in syrup form, which tasted like rotten bananas in milk. I developed an impressive gag reflex—even today, I cannot drink milk by itself or eat ripe bananas—so she started giving the antibiotic to me in pill form: white ovals, huge for my small throat. I would have to work up to swallowing them, like a horse attempting a jump: hold my breath, have a huge glass of water on hand, swallow as quickly and strongly as possible.

At some point, I started to hide these pills in the chimney. My parents were always distracted at dinnertime, and it was easy to stand there, feeling the sharp edges of the rocks at my back, holding the glass of water, and finding a crevice to wedge the pill in, to push it down out of sight. There must have been scores of those pills stuffed in the chimney by the time I left, a tower of them. As far as I know, they might still be all there back in New Zealand, gently decaying. I would inspect them, once in a while, while I was also watching Dad make dinner. They would yellow. With time and moisture, the outside of the pill would peel up away from its edges like paper, exposing the dry cement-looking texture of the inside of the pill.

More than twenty years later, that chimney suddenly came to mind when I was watching Ingmar Bergman's film *The Virgin Spring* with my students. I had not thought about the antibiotics or the chicken, but then, in the first scene, I saw a young woman called Ingeri, barely an adult, bracing her forearms on some kind of counter and bending low to blow upon a fire pit. Her hair was a dark, untamed mass, her skin gleaming with grime. When she stood, we could see that she was heavily pregnant, and that she wore a sackcloth coat. She picked up a large cast-iron pot without flinching, and hooked it to hang over the fire. The pot wasn't one she could afford if she was wearing that coat. If you asked me why I avoided pregnancy in my twenties, it was precisely because of this kind of image: chained to the kitchen, nourishing others. Ingeri wandered the room, then finally paused at a narrow wooden pole by the fire, which she grabbed and pushed upward, letting in air. The post opened a hole in the roof, revealing the sky. This is a chimney before chimneys existed. She clutched at the wooden pole as if she were drowning, and called. "Odin, come," she says. "Odin, come. Come to my aid." Even without knowing who that was, my students immediately understood she was working in someone else's home, and looking for escape.

The film was made in 1960, but that year does not seem to matter on Bergman's farm in Sweden, which is set clearly in premodern times, and is based on a thirteenth-century folksong. Time folded in on itself in the classroom. With my students, I watched Ingeri set the bowls out, and pour a bucket of milk into a trough covered in branches. Somehow, we knew that these branches were there to catch the globules of fat. Somehow, we understood that the barrels were filled with flatbread and sealed with planks of wood and stones. Somehow, we understood the number of large sharp knives and the absence of any other form of cutlery, why the father of the family, Töre, sat on a large wooden armchair that had roughly carved heads on top; this was a throne for a man who is king of a valley, and no more. We recognized the dynamics of the meal in that household. This must be what it feels like to be French, I thought, and dimly understand Italian by virtue of a casual historical proximity, a kind of automatic logic to living. I knew this kitchen, this table, even if I didn't know it. I knew that chimney, even if my own was different. Looking at Ingeri, I felt an instinctual sense of translation. This kind of archetypal echo is precisely what Hillman would've noticed and appreciated. There are forms to living that predate and postdate us, and when they are presented to us with as much focus as Bergman's, we hear the echo, a call in the valley. I remembered the feel of the scoria rock on my fingers as I pushed one pill, then another, down into the darkness. I had escaped, but now I was so far from home.

Odin is the guide of souls. His name is etymologically related to fury, to excitation, to mind, to poetry. And he does come to Ingeri, first disguised as a toad, and then as a man with warts and an overly familiar manner, who lives in the forest in a cottage filled with magical objects. He is laughable, and hugely powerful. Ingeri also appears to escape—but the way she does it is by destroying Karin, the daughter of the family that Ingeri serves. They are the same age, but Karin is blonde, well-dressed, clean, and chatty, blithe in her privilege. Walking through the woods together, they are waylaid: Ingeri by Odin, and Karin by three goatherds, who rape and murder her. Ingeri arrives in time to witness it all, to pick up a rock to defend Karin—and then, to put the rock back down, and do nothing.

Today, our sense of Bergman's old-world inevitability has been suspended: the scale of punishment in the film is reserved for good art, but not our own lives. Maybe our forms of punishment have become subtler, more devious: more decorative. If Nancy Meyers remade *The Virgin Spring*, no one would die. Ingeri would get a makeover and learn to lighten up. The film's last scene would be a last supper in the forest: all of the characters, seated at an impeccably arranged table in a clearing and enjoying a meal, the camera panning up and down the table, lingering on each person's face, their talking and laughing, the toasting and small private asides. "Give us our daily bread!" someone would cry, and we would know that it was daily, that this was not a boast, and we would exit the cinema under our own dull sun, longing for water glasses that would refract light that way, for love all around. I could feel an almost barometric pressure change in the room when I watched Karin's rape and death with my students, but it was so difficult for them to stomach the equation: Ingeri's freedom for Karin's humiliation and pain. They didn't know what to do with it, and so they laughed at the awkwardness of

Karin's death scene, trying to turn Bergman into Meyers, trying to make these girls' loss and gain tolerable. They would not want to call to Odin: he was too much to bear.

My mother watches me read to Anika over Skype, and asks me if I remember her reading to me when I was a child. When I pick up a bowl in front of the computer screen, she tells me she used to have one like it. Every so often, I receive a packet in the mail: my clothes, which she has kept, and is now doling out as Anika grows. She delights in the echo and I understand why, even though it also feels claustrophobic. Her love for me has always felt overwhelming, even greedy. She resists Meyers and the horror of Bourdieu's predictability. She wants something else, something beyond the perfection of a space: she wants *me*. For a long time, I couldn't give it to her; I looked for chimneys, for ways to resist her. I left home at seventeen, moved cities, then countries. I invested my own desire for a home in objects, which is why if, on one of her visits, my mother were to admire one of my bowls—on the outside, the luminescent white of an oyster shell, and on the inside, a light yellow glaze—I would shrug noncommittally, as if it was no big deal, as if I had barely noticed it at all. Now that I have my own child to overwhelm, I remember myself, sitting at the table as a child, watching my mother pick at that chicken, the grease on her hands, indulging herself before she sat down to join us. *There*, I think. *There* is a flicker of the old magic, the recognition I feel watching that first scene in *The Virgin Spring*. Picking at the carcass, she sucked the grease off her fingers. Now I do the same thing, standing at the kitchen bench, my child at the table in front of me. We are tasting our fingerprints, too, the whorls of skin. This is an older form of domesticity which predates the ornamental—or maybe, a sense of the domestic that predates *upon* the ornamental, that hunts it. Home. It all breaks down one day. Home is where you do not know how to hold back.

WHEN ANIKA WAKES UP these days, she walks out of her bedroom, clutching Sheepie, and climbs onto the couch, settling in her favorite place, pulling the rug up. While I warm some milk on the stove, she sits, looking out at the garden, quiet, gazing up at the trees and the brightening sky. I pour the milk into her elephant cup, which has a silicone cap and a trunk from which to drink, and bring it to her. "Read," she says, lifting her current favorite book up to me, and I sit down, open the cover, and begin. Her eyes follow, her concentration flaring, leaping upward: I almost feel it, a steady fierce flame next to me. We read, adrift in time. It feels a world away from where I began when she was a baby—she can walk, I can leave her on the couch, we can read together—but the actions keep the same rhythm, just in a different key. This understanding of the domestic is antithetical to Meyers's homes, not accounted for by any of those PRIZMs or by Bourdieu, and only a little by Barthes. It is a vision I now cling to, fiercely. My kitchen is also no longer well-equipped, or clean. Small things are also broken. Anika drapes herself over my body, chortling with laughter as I pretend to eat her, snuffling her stomach. Right now, she delights in how much I want her. I delight in how much she wants me. I have learned my mother's passion, understand it now, and I also do not know how to hold back, though I am always, always, watching for signs of engulfment, and escape. These days, I almost feel sorry for Hillman; I don't think he could see what is happening in moments like these: the co-creation of ritual, the inscribing of the eidetic. "Tell me a story," Anika says to me, and I watch the satisfaction in her eyes when I begin; the knowledge that I will begin by noticing what is not right, what has fallen, and what has to be made right. The scenes of my imagination are not estranged: if anything, they are *more* embodied than they've ever been. They are just harder to write down.

Whenever Anika walks into the room, the writing of this book stops. Her needs will continue to displace mine for a while longer, though the balance is shifting day by day, year by year. But if the child is equivalent with imagination, the mother's language frays into poetry, into elliptical phrases, line breaks you can almost see: hypotheticals and private jokes, murmurings, questions, resolutions. I used to think of time as a river, and I would swim along in it happily enough, moving with the current, which felt fairly constant: I could guess its velocity. Now, time is akin to that narrow patch of sand in between the waves and farther up the beach, where the sand is heaped and loose and deep. Walking along a beach, you try to find the hard stretches, the places where your feet firmly strike and you can move swiftly along. But every so often, you hit a sudden wetness or dryness, and your foot sinks, your body tilts, and another ratio of effort to velocity reveals itself. It becomes an art, a pleasure and frustration, trying to gauge by sight alone what the next step will feel like. With a child, my foot suddenly sinks: ten minutes becomes an age. A year is a blur. I have no constant velocity. I have become a time traveler, with little control over it. I am learning to accept this new rhythm that was always there.

Unlike most other cells in the body, the egg cell does not renew itself every seven years; oocytes mature, but they are not replaced. The eggs I was born with are the oldest cells in my body, which means my mother was born with the egg that I would one day develop from. In turn, the oocyte that will develop into any child Anika might choose to have (of her own genetic material) is already tucked away inside of her. It feels vertiginous knowing that half of my genetic material has been alive twice as long as I have, and that the egg that produced Anika has also been alive since before I was born. Biological mothers are threaded like daisy chains into and through their children, and their children into them. Both mother and child escape their life span, spill past the years declared on birth certificates and death certificates, but the child is not quite timeless, nor eternal. Nothing is timeless, but timeless isn't praise, as Hillman would appear to assume. A child resists any effort to make it time-bound, and the mother will be happier if she accommodates some of the resistance. Her morality is a bricolage, a reconstitution of what the child wants, what she was taught, and what others are now telling her to do. Her sense of the future is not as important as it used to be, or perhaps, future, present, past seem more obviously, ineluctably intermingled. She knows there are things over which she has no control.

"Look!" Anika says, "the moon!" It's still there, faintly hanging on in the sky.

12

. . .

SNOWFLAKE

The refrain of others, when you are trying and failing to fall pregnant, is that you can always adopt. When I realized I might not be able to have biological children of my own, I looked into it too. I personally knew of many successful adoptions, where it was clear the child was benefiting from a stable, loving environment. Online, agencies were quick to reassure families of the humanitarian value of an adoption: Who *wouldn't* want to think that the pain of infertility can also translate to a kind of heroism? But I could also immediately see how logistically difficult and ethically suspect it was going to be. The more I read about the history of adoption in the United States, the more cautious I grew.

Adoption has always been American in the way the World Series is; no other country has been as relentless in finding new markets for children or in crafting a sense of moral justification for the practice. Evangelical Christianity, in particular, developed an "orphan theology" movement in the 1990s that figured adoption as a grounding metaphor for religious conversion in general. By adopting a child, you were bringing one more soul into God's fold. Where these children came from (the proportion of intercountry, private agency, kinship, tribal, and public agency adoptions) changed over time. At its height in 1970, there were 175,000 adoptions of children and infants in the United States. By 2001, the number had decreased by about 50,000, but international markets had moved in boom-bust cycles for some time: China (in the 1990s), then Guatemala (in the early 2000s), then Ethiopia, Ghana, Haiti. A distinct pattern emerged; countries would be "opened up," then trend toward scarcity as a nation's government began to recognize the possible coercion and corruption involved: in a country where the average monthly wage might be $35, the price of a child was $5,000. All of these "sending" nations had average annual incomes far below that of the United States, and even when the children were voluntarily surrendered by their mothers, it seemed a fine line between ethical adoption and economic coercion. There are, of course, a number of reasons why women give up children for adoption, but a particu-larly well-documented reason is because they cannot afford to feed the child. If that is the case, shouldn't the ethical imperative be to address a mother's economic circumstances, rather than to raise her child half a world away? Every country I've listed above has since moved to limit the practice of adoption from the United States.

Embryo donation seemed more promising. Right now, there are more than a million embryos frozen in labs across the United States. No one is quite sure how many there are—there is no legal obliga-tion to accurately report numbers—but even a conservative esti-mate would rival the population of San Diego. More aggressive hormone stimulation protocols in the 1990s resulted in couples banking not just one or two, but 10, 15, even 20 embryos. Whereas other countries have a time limit by which parents should decide whether they should be donated to science or to another couple (and if not, destroyed), there is no such time limit in the United States. Couples are often caught: if they can't bring themselves to have the clinic destroy them, neither is it always straightforward to donate their embryos to scientific research that they know will be ethically conducted. In the early 2000s, as cryopreservation techniques improved, a third option—embryo donation—became increasingly viable. Couples could decide to help out another woman suffering from infertility. A little more than a year ago, with my FSH levels, that would have been me.

The prospect not just of adopting a child at birth, but of giving birth to it, gestating it—for it to be yours in every epigenetic way but the actual chromosomal DNA—is alluring. There is no developmental catch-up, no new language to learn, no ruffling of cultural feathers. With embryo adoption, there is also less economic coercion; indeed, because implantation is cheaper than stimulation, it reverses socioeconomic currents of privilege. The wealthy are offering parenthood to those less well off. Any trauma associated with the adoptive experience appears minimized (though not negated). In the 1990s, Nancy Verrier, an adoptive parent and psychologist, argued that adoption was a fundamentally wrenching experience, regardless of how either parent or child thought it worked out. To her, the wound created in separating a biological mother from a child was "physical, emotional, psychological, and spiritual," felt on a "cellular" level. With embryo donation, the scale of separation was completely different; any primal wound was a few cells old, rather than a few days or years.

What interested me was how quickly evangelical Christianity reframed IVF (which was far from an acceptable practice in many

Christian circles, considered a meddling with a natural, God-determined order) to encourage "embryo adoption." This pivot occurred in the late 1990s, precisely when international markets for adoption were undergoing boom-bust cycles. In 1997, Ron Stoddart, the director of Nightlight Christian Adoptions, one of the largest adoption agencies in the United States, reached out to James Dobson, one of the more prominent public voices among the Christian evangelical right in order to talk about repositioning human embryo transfer (HET). The rationalization was elegantly simple. Embryo adoption was a chance to rescue those who had been abandoned, to save them from science: all those souls on ice, waiting to be resurrected or condemned. Nightlight called the frozen embryos "snowflakes"—as in, no two the same. If one were to rename embryo donation as adoption, one could also indirectly reclassify three-day-old embryos as children, a not insignificant victory for the anti-abortion movement. Dobson was receptive to the idea, and so Stoddart went on to develop a strikingly similar process for embryo adoption as Nightlight followed for standard adoptions, instituting home visits, matching procedures, and counseling.

The effects of this are obvious decades later. In Nightlight's annual reports, there is barely any difference between how the adoption of a child and the adoption of an embryo is described. The rhetorical cadence in all the stories is strikingly similar: each family explains the reasons for their infertility, and isolates the moment when adoption was laid on their heart and when God revealed to them their mission. They rationalize the waiting, application process, and money; God would not have given them this weight if he thought they could not bear it. At the same time, God also resolved various difficulties, pushing through tests and paperwork. I read year after year of these reports, marveling at the syntax: each sentence leaned forward in its eagerness, meaning spilling from one clause onto the next, moving at speed toward the *fait accompli*: "She cried for 2 months every night from 8–12 and the whole time we were just thankful to God that we had her." The children needed love, and they had love to give, and all of this was a referred or echoed image of cosmic Love, a force that animates the world, as physically pervasive as air. These stories were often accompanied by a photo of the smiling family on a picnic blanket or in a park or in front of their house. Their certainty was unsettling.

In these embryo adoptions, the donating couple decides who gets their embryos. They can decide if the adopting couple needs to be married, and can refuse to accept single adopters or gay couples. They can require that the adopting couples be Christian. They can decide what state to adopt *to*, or if the adopting couple needs to be readers or play sports. When I started to draft my own profile, before I was able to conceive, I grew worried. Though the number of embryo donation agencies using more-inclusive language has increased in the past decade, many of them remain explicitly Christian. How on earth was I going to persuade any of these people to give *me* an embryo? How would I be able to write a story for their newsletter and match that syntax without feeling like a skeptical con? My ways of rationalizing my infertility were far too complicated. I had no idea of what kind of family I'd pose on that blanket. I strongly resented that I would have to be a supplicant.

IN THE NINETEENTH CENTURY, a number of men worked on atlases of human embryology which also required persuading people to give them embryos. One of the most well-known was Wilhelm His Sr., in Leipzig, Germany, who developed the microtome, a machine that sliced flesh (hardened with acids and salts) into very thin cross-sections that could then be fixed on slides. These slices allowed for an understanding of minute distinctions between different kinds of tissue—between, for example, epithelium, which lines cavities and covers surfaces of organs and the body, and endothelium, which lines the insides of blood vessels. Using this new technique, His prepared an atlas of human embryology by comprehensively documenting twelve human embryos that were between 2 and 8.5 weeks old. It took him years to assemble this collection; he had relied on colleagues across Europe who had sent him specimens, and which he named using the doctor's initials, or the city in which they resided. As a result, he worked with Lg, Bl, R, BR3, B, A N, S1, Sch, S2, Zw, and Lo.

In 1884, the American doctor Franklin Mall traveled to Germany, and ended up studying under His. Mall was also entranced by the microtome's revelations: embryos had been collected and dissected for the past century, but with this new technology you could now see inside the embryo with the clarity of a stained-glass window. Wilhelm His was focusing on the development of the nervous system, and was able to track, almost week by week, how embryonic nerve fibers developed. The meticulous description of development was a decisive turn away from preformist accounts of conception in the seventeenth century. Mall decided he needed to start a collection of his own. When he returned to the United States in 1886 (with two embryos given to him by His), Mall continued to expand his collection, placing advertisements in a number of medical journals, and eventually writing to more than half of the doctors in the United

States and abroad, offering to send them containers and covering all of their shipping costs. In a paper published in 1917, the year of his death, he noted that his collection contained approximately 2,000 embryos, and that it was increasing at the rate of 400 a year. Four years before, he had obtained the first of a series of grants that resulted in the formation of the Carnegie Institution of Washington's Department of Embryology, which would house his collection. By 1944, the collection was more than 9,000: the largest in the world.

Mall referred to his embryos by number; his correspondence with other doctors sounds like he could have been discussing plant and fruit seeds. To one doctor, thanking him for his continued involvement, he acknowledged that "we owe to your kindness specimens no. 21, 50, 439, 449, 460, 472, 481 and 486."

These are difficult numbers to comprehend, not simply because of the sheer number of specimens, but because the stories of the women from whom these embryos were removed have been so thoroughly erased. On rare occasion, the correspondence would mention the circumstances by which an embryo was obtained: the woman's age, the date of collection, and the cause (autopsy, hysterectomy, abortion, early labor). But *why* or how any of this had happened was considered irrelevant. In a 1904 textbook, J. Playfair McMurrich described the youngest embryo then known to (American) embryologists by noting it was "taken from the uterus of a woman who had committed suicide one calendar month after the last menstruation, and it measured about 1 mm in diameter." There was no speculation as to whether the pregnancy and the suicide were related.

In her book *Icons of Life*, the medical anthropologist Lynn M. Morgan attempted to reconstruct the narrative of one of the women from whom a Carnegie embryo, specimen 836, came. In Mall's records, Specimen 836's mother's name was listed as Mrs. R, a twenty-five-year-old woman from western Virginia who had undergone a hysterectomy, the standard treatment then for suspected fibroid tumors. (She had discovered a lump in her abdomen weeks earlier.) When her surgeon operated on her in Baltimore, he discovered the embryo, and sent the entire uterus to Mall, who was very pleased: the embryo was in near-perfect condition and one of the smallest he had received. With genealogical assistance, Morgan traced Mrs. R back to her town in western Virginia. It turned out she was not Mrs. but Miss (many maternity hospitals in the early twentieth century refused to treat unmarried women). Morgan ended up visiting Mrs. R's town, and tried to find her grave at the local cemetery. She could find Mrs. R's parents, brother, and sister, but there was no trace of Mrs. R's own grave, and no more information about her life. Only her embryo had entered the historical record: posed, drawn, photographed, and modeled on numerous occasions, all without Mrs. R even knowing it existed. In turn, Mrs. R's own existence was proved by her embryo *not* being born. In her book, Morgan movingly describes how, in her car, she circled and circled the cemetery, unable to leave, "increasingly distressed to think that Carnegie no. 836 was all that remained of her."

Morgan is absolutely correct to grieve. I grieve. And yet, as a potential embryo adopter, I found that instinctively, I also did not want to know much about the woman and man from whom a donated embryo might come. I worried their story would not align with mine. I worried they would want something different for it. The possibility of my interconnectivity was overwhelming. I knew this was a knee-jerk reaction, and one I wasn't proud of: it seemed entirely similar to an assimilationist ideology that had dogged adoption practices throughout the twentieth century. The swiftness with which I recategorized the ethical value of a narrative interested me.

Though it is not necessarily a widely acknowledged fact, it appears that embryo donation or adoption is not as popular an option as Christian adoption agencies hoped or predicted. Some studies estimate the percentage of couples willing to donate their embryo as between 5 percent and 10 percent. Regardless of religious affiliation, to those who have undergone IVF, who have made such an effort to create life, it can seem perverse to give it away. Each harvested egg is counted with excitement, each fertilized embryo celebrated. The industry is eager to sentimentalize this moment of potential because it provides the emotional payoff for a stressful experience. For couples, these embryos are joint property, the expression of a future together. The photos they bring home from the embryology lab are as concrete and emotionally significant as a joint mortgage or a marriage certificate. To do *anything* with the embryo other than attempt implantation requires an awkward conceptual pivot, a reframing of the significance of what has just been endured. What obligation do you have to an embryo that, if gestated and born, would be a sibling to your own children? What if the family you donated the embryo to mistreated that child? What responsibility remains; shadows you, like a dream?

Doubts or questions like these are not easily conveyed in the newsletters of adoption agencies, and so in order to understand more about what the experience felt like, I spoke to ten women across the United States in 2016, after Anika was born, who either worked for embryo adoption agencies or were embryo adopters or donors. Half were from the Midwest. I was very curious to hear from the women what it had been like to make their decision. Was there any trauma at all? Had they told their children? Had their thinking changed as time had passed? Did they still feel like they had saved a soul (if they had thought that in the first place)? The months in which I spoke to them spanned the birth of Anika and also happened to coincide with the 2016 presidential election in the United States, and Donald Trump's win over Hillary Clinton. We did not talk about politics, though I guessed theirs, and I'm sure they guessed mine. An awkward coincidence at this time was that the go-to dismissal of liberal voters grieving the election results "snow-flakes": here I was, asking about these women's snowflakes when I was the snowflake. We persisted. They were willing to talk to me because they knew I had experienced infertility. They knew that I knew how it felt to not be able to have a child. They also knew that I had two snowflakes of my own, from my first round of IVF.

Most of them had not told people about their experience with embryo donation or adoption. One woman went so far as to only tell me the state she lived in, rather than the town or city. They were sometimes protective because they had not told their children of the fact; other times, it was known inside the family, but not outside it. I asked the women who had adopted embryos if they found them-selves thinking about that fact much, and nearly all said they didn't. It was impossible, they said, *not* to feel like the child was utterly theirs the more their lives were upended by it: the sleepless nights, rushed days, the whirlwind of love and labor. More than one noted that the child looked uncannily like them. They preferred to forget about the adoption, to move on. Some had attempted "open" em-bryo adoptions, which meant meeting the family of their donated embryo, once it was born. One or two families celebrated holidays like Thanksgiving together; they wanted to give the children a sibling experience. But others described losing contact with the adoptive family. It was too painful, they said—either for them, or the other family. They didn't agree on parenting strategies. Only one woman said she still thought about the genetic difference, and this was because she chose embryo donation deliberately: alcoholism ran in her family, and she wanted to avoid it. She celebrated saving them from her own genetic legacy. I heard in all of their voices a decisiveness, a slicing and separation of all possible futures away from this one. I had a hard time deciding if this decisiveness had been sharpened by shame. There was nothing shameful about the practice—and yet, here I was, waiting for a call from an unlisted number, from a woman who really did not want to tell me her name. We could call her Mrs. R.

While I was talking to these women, I also decided to go online and reactivate a dating profile. At that point nearly all of my daily actions had no seeming end, and although the repetition was important, there were days where it also felt corrosive, like a mild acid. As a series of firsts (first conversations, first kisses, etc.), dating appeared to me to have an alkaline, neutralizing effect. On my profile, I did not state I was a mother: I could barely say the word out loud to friends. I clicked through the first ten matches the algorithm gave me, and Zac's was probably one of the first five I saw. I thought, *He'll do*. I agreed on a time and place, marveling that this was what it felt like to actually date with no expectations.

Zac turned out to be easy to talk to, quick-witted, and slow to stress. We talked for a few hours, and then I rushed home to breast-feed. On the second date, he made a crack about women with strollers, and I knew I had to say something. I was visibly, audibly awkward, apologizing profusely. "Well that's a bombshell," he said. He and I were both traveling over the next month, and I suggested we both take some time to think about what to do next. When we returned to New York, we fell into the rhythm of seeing each other once or twice a week. He didn't meet Anika for another two months, and I made it completely clear that I was not expecting him to behave like a parent. Anika already had a father. It helped that Zac was not particularly interested in children; it wasn't that he disliked them, but he had never wanted a family in that way. We were both good at compartmentalizing our lives. Shahzad was sleeping on the couch in my apartment, and would continue to do so for the next two years. He and Zac learned to maneuver around each other. Shortly after Anika was born, Shahzad also reconnected with Gyda, with whom he had partnered after our relationship. They saw each other on tour, in Iceland, occasionally in New York. When everyone was in town, we'd have dinner together: Anika sitting in her seat, surrounded by four adults, each from a different part of the world, talking and eating. When I went back to work, I hired two women, Julia and JoyAnn, who also each looked after Anika for two days a week. When my aunt and uncle came to visit, they reported back to my father that the apartment seemed like Grand Central Station, but that everyone seemed remarkably calm about it all. I think Zac and I continued to see each other because we liked each other a great deal, and because we both instinctively agreed that the relationship needed a light touch: it seemed highly unlikely it was going to work, so we simply enjoyed it.

When Anika was about nine months old, my milk supply halved in one day. That night, I looked up the causes, and realized that I could be pregnant. This time around, the pregnancy test was unbearably quick: positive. The dismay and shock I felt was nauseating. *So this is what it feels like,* I remember thinking. This is what it means to *fall* pregnant. The vertigo of that realization, the panic: the whole thing appeared to be a once-in-a-million biological rimshot. I was not ready for this. I wasn't supposed to be *able* to do this.

Anika was barely sleeping for five hours at a stretch at night, and my relationship with Zac was four months old. I had a full-time job, and was living half a world away from any family. Though I was handling one baby well, I did not have the financial resources, the stamina, or the emotional support to have a second. It was all too complicated. Zac didn't want one either. I thought it very likely that our relationship would not withstand a child. I would end up coparenting one child, and single-mothering another. The panic felt like a sudden flash fire: this was not possible. Any hard-won sense of what pregnancy meant to me and my body was upended. For almost two years, I had thought of myself as infertile, or close to it. I had so focused on my FSH and AMH numbers that I overlooked the crucial point that all I needed was one good egg to fall pregnant. Now it was as if I had landed on a different planet, with differing ratios of gases and gravities, and I struggled to acclimate to this new conception of myself. I had passed through a two-week wait without knowing it. No one had seen inside me: I hadn't seen myself. Once again, I did not know what was happening to me, even though this time it was happening naturally. Ironically, it felt even *more* discontinuous as an experience. The conceptual whiplash of this still feels jarring to me, years later.

Usually, women approximately age a pregnancy by their last period, but because I was breastfeeding, my period had barely returned. Judging by the way the milk supply had suddenly halved, the pregnancy was recent. I rang an abortion clinic almost immediately. Having spent months researching embryos, I understood more about cell development, and had developed my own moral limit, which was quite independent of any legal finding. I did not want to abort an embryo after the primitive streak, which was at about fifteen days old, and which marked the beginning of individual cellular development. I found a discreet office in midtown, the kind of place where they only ever had one patient at a time in the waiting room. Early abortion was all they did. I made an appointment for the next day. I couldn't afford to wait.

The ultrasound confirmed the pregnancy, and the fact that it was extremely early; in fact, so early that they wanted me to wait a week until it was clearer what they were excising: any embryo this small would be easier to miss. I lay on the table, not wanting to look at the screen, looking instead at the doctor, trying to explain how important it was to me that I do this now, and not wait a week. She nodded, understood, and informed her assistants. I had spent months desperately trying to gain one collection of cells, and here I was destroying another. I had burst into tears of joy when I had seen every ultrasound of Anika, and now I turned my head from the inky whiteness and blackness. It was too identical to be bearable. I was given pain relief, held Zac's hand, and quickly, within five minutes, it was done, the embryo scraped off the side of my uterus using a small suction tool. My body convulsed in a wave of cramps—but it was nothing, *nothing*, next to bringing a fetus to term and giving birth.

The next day, I went on the pill.

In another age, this embryo could have been sent to an institute, preserved and sliced. (My own would've been around the same age as Specimen 836.) It would have been registered under my doctor's name, and classified as belonging to one of twenty-three stages of embryonic and fetal development. My age might have been recorded, but the circumstances of the embryo's removal—which mean everything to me—would not. Historically, at least, my reasons for the abortion are not considered important, nor how significant the event was relative to the rest of my life, how it nestles in among other pains and joys.

It's now the case that images of hundreds of embryos from the Carnegie Collection of Embryology have been scanned and digitized, and are available online. There is a photograph of Specimen 836, curled into itself like a fiddlehead fern. There are reproductions of exquisite pen and ink drawings from the early twentieth century, key body parts labeled. There are photographs of a sectioned embryo in its sequence of slides, laid out like playing cards in a grid. There are awkwardly digitized 3D models, where you can rotate the embryo left and right, up and down, exploring its concavities as if you were playing a computer game. And there are "fly-through" videos, which have turned the sections into stop-motion films, an animation of what it looks like to move *through* an embryo. The flesh is stained pink and red, utterly abstract and as surreally absorbing as an early Len Lye film. An oval widens and lengthens. Different organs appear as landscape features, as tidal pools and underwater reefs, a Rorschach test in delicate pinks and reds. I can find out when the specimen was preserved, and what fixative was used. If it was sectioned, I will know whether the cut was transverse (cutting horizontally, as if you were slicing a pickle), coronal (vertically, dividing back from front), or sagittal (vertically again, dividing left from right). These images make it abundantly clear how complex and beautiful embryonic development is. If it is *not* my embryo, I am fascinated. We move from two cells to what looks like a slender, vertically shaped jellyfish, just a wisp of a thing, a smear of tissue, to a compact creature, tail rounded, bulbous forehead tucked down, its lines as compact and brief as a primitive wooden amulet; to arm and leg stubs growing like buttons; and finally, a fish-eyed alien with black eyes. This is just the first two months. Looking at these images, I feel the relief of sitting on this side of the screen with coffee and the sounds of the building around me. The embryos radiate intent. It is hard to remember they are dead, though their isolation is stark: they are not photographs in situ in a body or uterine tissue, but float, permanently detached, folded away from the bodily experiences of pregnancy, like a pressed flower. If this is my embryo, I feel great pity. It violates what feels instinctively private. I toggle back and forth in my mind, trying each point of view on for size: mine, not mine. Mine, not mine. This is the difference between being the bottle, and looking at it. To confront one's aspectual morality is rarely a comfortable thing.

I stopped talking to the women who had adopted embryos, or who had facilitated adoptions. I felt ashamed that I had so quickly recategorized the life in my body. I assumed they wouldn't understand it, and wouldn't agree with my own assessment of their ambivalence, their own silences on the phone line. There were no easy rhetorical forms within which to express my abortion. Doubt was not to be trusted. Despite the triumphant Christian rhetoric of embryo adoption, despite the fact that we live in a culture where the testimonial has become a genre of daytime TV, we are still so cautious when it comes to the embryo. There is a tradition of silence. Not writing about an embryo, or about women's reproductive choices, renders those decisions dark matter in our lives. We only sense its weight by how other planetary bodies move. Circumspection ends up as excision. I thought about the rhetorical forms that might govern my story, what rhythm there was between uncertainty and moral clarity. I wondered if my sentences leaned forward, or backward, where meaning accrued. I did not tell many people about this abortion. Writing an account of one's embryos has fixed, like His's techniques, an experience that has also continued to change shape in my mind. There are two representations: how I think of it now, and how I narrated it to myself then. The discrepancy isn't surprising, but its existence does make me cautious. If it is my embryo. If it is not. I am capable of recalibrating my world with a collection of cells that is barely the size of one of these letters.

I HAVE AVOIDED talking about Shahzad for the most part here, mostly fearing other people's judgment, but having gone through an unwanted pregnancy, I now see how significant he is. I had thought of my decision to co-parent with him as one born of necessity, but my decision making was more precise than I initially cared to admit.

Shahzad had a very different childhood than I did, though we're both children of doctors. For decades, his mother worked as a psychiatrist in a number of institutions across Pennsylvania and New York State, and Shahzad spent years of his life growing up in houses on the grounds of each institution. As a Pakistani-American kid growing up in small-town Pennsylvania, he would've attracted racist comments regardless, but he also had ectodermal dysplasia, which makes him look very different: he has an unusually shaped nose, chin, and brow. He has no sweat glands, and his skin is as smooth as paper. He has barely any hair, only wisps on his head. He was born with only three teeth in his jaw, and learned to talk with only upper dentures. He has never had lower dentures. His limbs and fingers seem slightly longer than anyone else's, as if he were a figure from a Mannerist painting come to life. He was also born with three fused bone plates in his skull, and so, when he was only a few months old, had artificial sutures inserted into his skull so his brain had room to expand as it grew. For a year or so as a child, he lived in a bubble at the hospital, almost blind. He cannot regulate his own body's temperature without sweat glands, and as a child, had to learn forms of self-regulation that ruled out sports, dancing, or simply hanging out on hot days with no water or air conditioning nearby. At school assemblies, people refused to sit next to him in all four directions: the hall might have been full, but there was always an empty seat behind, in front, and to the left and right of him. As a child, he begged his parents to move to a city. He says he made his first non-familial friends at college. When you google his name, the "related searches" at the bottom of the page nearly always include mention of an accident, a fire, and his skull.

Every so often, someone will politely ask me about genetic testing. Inheritance patterns for ectodermal dysplasia are more complicated than most people know. We determined that I was not a carrier for it, but any female child of mine would be, and up to 70 percent of female carriers can exhibit mild symptoms of the condition. Shahzad's mother is also a carrier, and she has no symptoms of which I'm aware—and when Anika was born, she also showed no symptoms. With time, a few traits have emerged. She is missing one tooth in her upper jaw and one on the bottom. When she's hot, her nose tends to sweat profusely. No one looking at her would diagnose her with the condition, nor has it interfered at all with her ability to lead a very active life. It could also be possible that these tiny signs are not signs of ectodermal dysplasia at all: my mother is also missing a tooth in her upper jaw. These details are so minimal that it is tempting to overlook any diagnosis altogether, which we have essentially done. Like many other people who have been categorized or diagnosed as exhibiting a disorder, Shahzad is skeptical of any label's usefulness in doing anything other than establishing normative models for living. His power as an individual is closely intertwined with his condition. At a young age, he understood others' capacity for cruelty. He met doctors who treated him with compassion and love. He saw how social arrangements could be deeply provisional. He would not have been able to act as he has throughout his life without this knowledge, no matter how unsettling it was. As we proceeded through IVF, we saw for ourselves the pressures to select "healthy" embryos through pre-implantation genetic diagnosis (PGD or PIGD), which is when a fragment of an embryo is tested for chromosomal irregularities before it is implanted in the womb. It was a gentle pressure, but persistent, and usually framed in terms of implantation success. We chose not to do PGD for our first round of IVF because we did not want to tacitly accept that Shahzad's condition was something to be avoided, and also because we knew that any child's symptoms would be significantly fewer than his. For the second round of IVF, we had less choice: the embryologist thought it better odds for implantation if we implanted those embryos at three days old, rather than five, which meant that PGD couldn't be performed. We chose to take the risk.

I am uncomfortable writing at length about Shahzad's ectodermal dysplasia; day-to-day, it's not something we really talk about.

And yet I think he would agree with Mitchison's spacewoman and her interest in biological cause and social effect, in how our physiological structure directs our cognitive and moral frameworks. When I first met Shahzad in New York, he was a downtown improvisational musician, and worlds away from where he grew up, as well as from the wishes of his parents, who badly wanted him to become a doctor. All told, he *loves* hospitals; as soon as he's in one, you can see him visibly relax. These are people who have always tried to make him better, have always tried to relieve his suffering. He understands how to get their attention. But he had spent most of his life ignoring the limitations placed on him by his health and had developed a profound skepticism toward any sense of a social contract. He does not believe in statistics, only in the existence of outliers. He carries a guitar everywhere he goes, and feels no concern about playing it, regardless of any constrained silence. When I first met him, he appeared *sui generis*, more like an alien than a man able to stretch any moment—a dinner, the line at the DMV, a boat ride—into a completely different set of dimensions. To someone who had spent her life quietly trying to do the same thing without anyone watching, it was both horrifying and liberating to watch other people watch him, to see him lean into the stares of others and not break. Being with him felt like hacking into life: all the stuff you weren't supposed to do, you could now do.

We were together as a couple for seven years, which felt long enough for me to understand what wouldn't change about him. For me, seeing is knowing. For him, knowing has always been sound and touch, the almost-electricity generated by presence. When he plays the bass, he often turns his head to one side, but it is not a cocking so much as a slow nodding, an agreement: yes, this is right. He is listening to the room rather than the music. When I started to consider IVF, he seemed a great fellow traveler for the journey. I could rely on him to not be scornful or intimidated by the medicine. Even if he had had to undergo the IVF injections and surgery himself, he would have still categorized it as a minimal intrusion. His skepticism of statistics and the social contract was a useful counterbalance to my own tendencies, as was his commitment to improvisation in pretty much every aspect of his life. I knew he would teach a child to not be afraid of the world, to step forward rather than hang back. I knew a child of his would grow up feeling comfortable with change and difference.

I also knew that we would never get back together. It was stabilizing to understand that he was not my emotional center, and I was not his. Most people would consider this crazy talk, and assume that it is dangerous for a family if the parents' desires are directed outward at other people, rather than inward. But for me it felt far more destabilizing to expect that one person *could* be everything. I am sure this intuition was formed when my parents separated when I was eighteen years old, and no distinction was made at the time between their marriage and our family, no discussion of how one might end and the other continue. My parents have not seen or spoken with each other more than a few times in the two decades since. The four of us have not gathered together once. I don't write this to embarrass them, but to point out how my own choices were an extension of this disruption. I created a family that doesn't require marriage or a mate. It is now a built-in feature of my life that my family is distinct from any sexual relationship I might have; if the latter ends, the former will always continue. I will never have to negotiate that separation because it has already happened.

When Anika turned two years old and was able to climb out of her crib by herself, she started to regularly make her way from her bedroom to mine in the middle of the night. I'd hear the padding rush of her feet and sit up, calling softly to her. She would come to the bed, and I would lift her up and into the bed where she lay between Zac and me, holding Sheepie, delicately pulling at his tail, eyes open, watching the shadows on the ceiling cast by the streetlamp through the shutters. Slowly, her lids would lower. Her breathing would shift gear. In those moments, wrapped in the comforter and the echo of sleep, I felt like the three of us were in a small boat in the vast ocean, pulling at our oars together in synchronizing breath. This is what a marriage or partnership might feel like, I'd think: the circling of prairie wagons, a thick distinction between private and public. I sensed how that scale of commitment to another person had a catalytic force, allowing a new compound to form. I worried that this scale was missing from my life.

Zac and I continued to take things very slowly, and that conferred its own stability. He barely looked after Anika by himself for the first two years. He did not move in until she was four. His relationship with Anika often seems more like a sibling's than a stepparent's; they both delight in annoying each other. I am only just starting to understand the depths of his own habits, as he is with mine. He is more socially constrained; though his father is Puerto Rican, Zac looks and sounds as white and as English as they come, and he spent his youth partying and working in PR agencies in London. He loves good food, good wine, good books, and is quietly unembarrassed about arranging his life around these enjoyments. I love him more and more, and I see how my earlier intuition was correct; he is too set in his ways for me to have done anything other than the lion's share of parenting if we'd had a child, and I would've resented that enough to make it difficult for me to be with him.

When I was pregnant with Anika, I would have never guessed that this was what family would look like. Shahzad has since married Gyda, and she loves Anika dearly. Anika loves her right back. Many times now, Shahzad, Gyda, Zac, and I have gone on holiday together with Anika. We talk multiple times a day, live blocks from one another. At school, she has pictures of all of us in her cubby. Shahzad and I disagree on a number of things, some more serious than others: appropriate car seat installation, food, naps, routines. At times, it is maddening. But our oppositional qualities have also remained generative. I am proud when I see elements of him in Anika; a look, a chortle, a wiggly sidewalk dance. At its best, this web of affection feels clannish, improvisational, and joyful. Anika has developed her own particular games and rituals with each person, and the tiny permutations of each day create an evolving lexicon. Our parenting has less certainty than the way my parents did it, but it also has less pained obligation. Shahzad and I are the sun and moon to Anika, but she is not very preoccupied by the ways in which we do or do not orbit one another. The whole thing might feel a little more provisional, but it does not feel uncertain. We are adamant in our love.

Our two snowflakes from the first round of IVF remain at the clinic, cryopreserved. Shahzad does not want a second child: he loves Anika so much, but it has been an enormous disruption to his career and his freedom of movement. Zac does not want me to use one of these embryos for reasons most people would find obvious. I vacillate, as always: there are days I think Anika and I could handle the complexity, and days I think we couldn't. Every six months, I receive a bill for the cryopreservation costs. Even after all I have been through, I cannot bring myself to destroy them, or give them away. My sense of family is always changing, and I am afraid that writing about it—like my abortions—will preserve something that shouldn't be hardened. I am afraid I will jinx it, inadvertently describing the loopholes through which disintegration and dismay can slip. And yet I am also mindful that the only way to widen our sense of alternative family structures or reproductive desire is to account for our own lives as precisely as we can. Parenthood turns out to be a series of ages rather than a single era; what I am like as the mother of a four-year-old is different from what I am like when she was five months old. Noticing this, I have grown more patient. I am waiting for it to become clear what I need to do.

13

THROUGH THE HATCH

In 2008, the anthropologist Sarah Franklin visited Guy's Hospital in London to conduct field research at a lab recently constructed using British government funding, which had been designed to bring new reproductive technologies and stem-cell research together: in the same building, on the same floor, couples could donate spare or clinically nonviable embryos to research that would take place on the other side of the wall. The pipeline from infertility treatment to stem-cell research had been shortened to become, literally, a hole in the wall. Franklin included a picture of the hatch in her book.

Whereas the other chapters in her book *Biological Relatives: IVF, Stem Cells, and the Future of Kinship* read as a more conventional academic text, written in the third person, Franklin kept her visit to Guy's Hospital in the form of first-person field notes. She is meticulous in describing what she sees. A postdoctoral researcher called Emma helps Franklin through two air locks, where she removes her clothes and puts on a new sterile lab suit and plastic clogs. In the lab, Vicky, another postdoctoral researcher, shows her the feeder cells they are using to grow human stem-cell lines. Franklin's notes are patient and pragmatic, which allows the quotidian nature of this technology to become fully apparent. Every day, Vicky and Emma tend their stem-cell colonies in the way a gardener might cultivate a patch of land. These women have learned to sense when their colonies are "happy," or when something's wrong. They intuit "when to cut them, when to leave them, when to add a bit of extra something in the media." None of it is overtly mechanized; Franklin watches one woman tease apart a colony of cells by hand, using a micropipette to passage sections of a cell colony into new "wells" to create room. "Even in this ultramodern lab, full of noisy respiring machinery," Franklin writes, "there is also a profound sense of craft." People still blow their own glass pipettes. Their equipment functions as an extension of their own senses; workers use a microscope as casually and as fluidly as you would a pair of glasses. The laboratory technicians and staff are mostly women. Franklin describes the banter, watching the way they "inhabit each other's space like the long-term, cloistered crew of a submarine."

Though Franklin doesn't explicitly note it, her description is pointedly at odds with the opening tour of the Central London Hatchery and Conditioning Centre in Huxley's novel *Brave New World*. Both books begin with an office building in London, and both books describe a process of cell growth which challenges our own expectations of reproductive singularity, but there the similarities end. In Huxley's novel, cell duplication is highly mechanized, proudly Fordist, a conveyor belt of reproduction. The Director is speaking only to men. Cell growth is not done by keeping cells "happy," but by stressing them: Huxley modeled his cloning process on parthenogenesis, in which an egg experiences some kind of chemical stress and divides without fertilization. The Director proudly speaks to his students: the process they've developed can produce ninety-six twins from a single embryo. In his words, we are far from the "old viviparous days," when an egg could only and sometimes accidentally divide into two or three. What seems comical now is how *low* the Director's numbers are: the researchers at Guy's Hospital are passaging *millions* of cells, all generated from embryonic donation. In *Brave New World*, examination has a cost. "Embryos are like photograph film," a worker says, pushing the door open to the Embryo Store: "They can only stand red light."

For centuries, looking inside involved death. William Harvey—the first person to discover that the heart was responsible for circulating blood around the body—did so through the live vivisection of animals. Like Karl Ernst von Baer, he often used dogs, but needed to keep them briefly alive, revealing the chest cavity and the beating heart before puncturing the muscle to show the considerable volume of pressurized blood. This was not an occasional torture. He had a dissection room in his house, stocked with a wide range of animals waiting to die: bottles and buckets containing toads, crabs, shrimp, whelks, oysters, and fish of various kinds; lizards, tortoises, serpents, fowl, pigeons, geese, rabbits, and mice scurrying around or lying lazily in cages and hutches; larger kennels for the sheep, pigs, and dogs. His laboratory—and many others—must've resembled a painting by Chaïm Soutine, pulsing with death and curiosity, with the delighted awareness that one is alive to witness what cannot witness itself. Harvey was exemplary in his efforts, but far from unusual. For a moment, think of the charnel heap that has advanced our looking: the thousands of unnamed women dissected, the countless jars of blood withdrawn and received. Think of Sims's

experiments on his enslaved patients. *If you can see it, you can fix it.*
Think of Nilsson's photographs for *Life* magazine, or Flanagan's reproduction of Hooker's dying fetuses. Think of the embryos and
blastocysts meticulously recorded by Purdy, Edwards, and Steptoe,
when they were years away from implantation. Think of Shettles's
Ovum Humanum. Think of His's microtome, and Mall's collection of
nine thousand embryos. Even the development of medical imaging
itself through the nineteenth and early twentieth century extracted
a price. Thomas Edison delayed development on his X-ray machine
because one of his workers, Clarence Madison Dally (who had the
habit of routinely X-raying both his hands), had to have both arms
amputated and eventually died. The side effects—burns, radiation
poisoning, and cancer—were obvious, as were the side effects of ra-
dionuclides, which, when injected, helped visualize blood vessels,
digestive and gastrointestinal systems, bile ducts and gallbladders.
Late–twentieth century medical visualizing technologies like ultrasound and laparoscopy are revolutionary precisely because their
physical impact on the body is a difference in kind rather than
degree.

The looking described in the lab at Guy's Hospital is strikingly
benign. Though the embryos from which these stem cells have been
extracted will not become human beings, their cells continue to
grow, duplicate: this is life, but on a different plane of human existence altogether. Looking is designed to aid growth, to monitor it.
In general, we appear to have shifted, in the late twentieth century,
toward different intimacies of looking at bodies that also have
different relationships to time. There is a distinct shift between
understanding anatomy as a two-dimensional static image, as an
etching or illustration or slide, and understanding the body through

ultrasound and camera as a body *in* time. The latter kind of looking feels epistemologically different. If the experience of infertility tends to halt a woman's sense of time, to place her in suspension, in an airless room—waiting, always waiting—video might open a window. Video is less of a separation than a branching, a wormhole that briefly constructs a parallel reality. Our body has always been moving, growing. Think of the roving obsessiveness of your tongue in the dentist's mouth mirror; rarely do we get to see that corporeal stubbornness. Here are your follicles, twitching, again, and again, and again. A fiber-optic cable will be threaded up through your vagina and in toward your ovary. Your eggs will be examined by microscope. If they fertilize, they will be looked at by a team of people you don't know before they are even three days old. Life doesn't begin in the secrecy of the body now—it begins out on the open plains of the petri dish, but these latter forms of image making underscore the present, rather than the past. They might diagnose my discontinuities of experience, might tell me what I do not know, but they're also a reminder of my stubborn, twitching continuance.

Of everything I have read, Franklin's account comes closest to achieving some kind of paradigm shift in the conception of human life, partly because these sections are so rhetorically rooted in the robust tradition of first-person empirical observation in Western science. But now, rather than men working alone, we have teams of women in labs, carrying dishes of cells cautiously, like bowls of hot soup. Franklin's photographs in the book are selfies with lab technicians, a pile of laboratory-only flat shoes. The incubators look like fridges. Franklin's focus is meant to challenge the old chestnut that technology is inhuman—the entire lab, she points out, is a giant human petri dish in more ways than one—but for me, what is more striking about her descriptions is her sense of domesticity. These women are delicately building a scaffold of cells that goes on and on, far beyond the bodies of their makers, who might be drinking a cup of tea in Aylesbury, the baby sleeping in the other room. Stem-cell production appears as a counterbalance to dissection and death: rather than fixing and staining, rather than a mechanized system of production, we also have cultivation and growth. This is a lab where the body is a dynamic process that does not seem to really stop, a place where we do not *have* to kill a cell to watch it divide, where cells that would not have developed into children are given the chance to replicate in an entirely new way. Indeed, the individual cell is not the significant unit of measurement. Though the hospital staff speak of the wonder of dealing with an almost literal distillation of life force, they do not talk about the cells as human or as containing a singular identity or consciousness.

This may sound too easy, too effortlessly a sequel to Mitchison's *Memoirs of a Spacewoman*. It's not that Franklin is optimistic about IVF or other new reproductive technologies. "As Foucault might have observed," she writes, "IVF is normal because it already belongs to techniques of normalization." It adds "a degree of flexibility to the reproduction of reproduction, while largely keeping the structure of bilateral biological kinship norms intact." It pretends to be the same and is not—and she sees this technological ambivalence as quietly destabilizing. She lists the "disjointed temporalities, jangled emotions, difficult decisions, unfamiliar procedures, medical jargon, and metabolic chaos" that IVF produces, the cognitive dissonance required in being encouraged to "believe you will succeed even though you will probably fail."

But she is optimistic about how we might reframe this knowledge, and turns to Donna Haraway and her now-iconic essay "A Manifesto for Cyborgs," to tease out this direction. Haraway's essay, published in 1985, is still an unnerving read today, precisely because she articulates a vision of the then-present that society has been unable to realize. Haraway argues that our "form of social existence has permanently displaced the dualisms of nature and science," that we are already (in 1985) "cyborgs, hybrids, mosaics, chimeras . . . There is no fundamental, ontological separation in our formal knowledge of machine and organism, of technical and organic." Because the old dualisms no longer apply for Haraway—and think of how excessively true this is today, in our age of smartphones, of operating systems that come with pictures of nature, of deepfakes and fitness watches—we can think instead of how the "common language" of a cyborg offers a way to reframe "intense pleasure in skill, machine skill" not as a "sin, but an aspect of embodiment." Writing this on a laptop, it is hard not to see the truth in her words. For Haraway, acknowledging how we might be both "animal and machine, who populate worlds ambiguously natural and crafted," might allow us to escape what Franklin paraphrases as "outdated organicist appeals to a pretechnologized nature or body."

It is very hard, when reading Haraway's encouragements, to *not* think of the magazines stacked in the waiting rooms of each IVF clinic I have visited, the endlessly rotating selection of lite reading that regularly celebrates natural births, natural bodies, and natural instinct. I think back to the day of my first retrieval, and my impulse, which felt a little odd at the time, to photograph these magazine covers. I thought I was capturing the banality of that day. I also think it was a protest that didn't know it was a protest: *these* are the guides they are providing me. This is what is on hand. Of course, it is more complicated; one of the magazines celebrated Caitlyn Jenner's then ongoing sex transition—but its newsworthiness was determined by precisely how "unusual" it was, and within the most well-known social media celebrity family in the United States at the time. The support for transition was prudishly prurient.

Franklin points out that an earlier draft of Haraway's "A Cyborg Manifesto," submitted to *Das Argument* (a German Marxist magazine), included comments on IVF and prenatal screening. These two technologies do not feature in the final version of the published essay. Haraway saw the potential of IVF to challenge the distinction between nature and science, but worried it could reinforce existing forms of inequality (which it has). She noted the technique was in its infancy ("a few hundred such babies are underway"), and described its potential, "about 35,000 babies per year" (now a considerable understatement). The future, she predicted, "was not bright"—she saw no reason why new reproductive technologies *wouldn't* develop through research on economically disadvantaged women ("for example the trials of the pill in Puerto Rico"). As long as it remained "within heterosexual, wealthy contexts," it would remain "conceived as a matter of private medical practice. . . . At present, IVF practice makes starkly clear class bias, heterosexism, and commodification of children in the social and technical systems critical to genetic engineering." In Haraway's subsequent draft, she left this section out, partly because it offered her no way out, no way to move toward a manifesto rather than a critique. IVF was a cul-de-sac, a catechism, a repetition of social forces she wished to disrupt. It did not point directly enough toward where she ultimately began her essay, which was her intention to blaspheme: "I know no better stance to adopt from within the secular-religious, evangelical traditions of United States politics. . . . Blasphemy protects one from the moral majority within, while still insisting on the need for community. Blasphemy is not apostasy." Her intention was to disrupt, all the while insisting on the continuity of her disruption, the way in which it did not constitute a new beginning, but a reframing of the past. She was in pursuit of a transgressive re-seeing, and IVF felt too conservative, too much a repetition rather than an alteration.

As Franklin notes, there is a "strange folding" of repetition involved in IVF, a turning back of meaning onto itself. Conceiving through IVF is not at all the same as conceiving through sex, but it is hard to know what to do with the phenomenological chasm and the promise of an identical outcome: a child. It could be said that this ambivalence extends to a basic ambiguity around the use of the word *reproduction*: we are not making copies of ourselves, but the word suggests we are. Regardless of where this ambivalence originates, the gap remains both narrow and deep, which makes it difficult to tease out the more radical potential of IVF. Our attempt to do so is often stymied by the ways in which multiple systems of regulation—capitalist, aesthetic, domestic—interpenetrate one another. IVF does not celebrate its ability to embroider upon one's cyborgian tendencies. It does not think in terms of kinship, in a centrifugal scaffolding of relation that might stretch and grow in multiple different directions, but instead focuses on celebrating the nuclearity of family, its centripetal force. If the IVF industry wanted to expand our understanding of kinship, there would be very different policies in place for single women who wished to conceive, as well as for trans, nonbinary, gay, and queer couples. There would be different policies on donor sperm. There would be a distinct effort to champion low-cost methods of IVF. Clinics would be interested in publicizing the diversity of their patients, as well as a diversity of opinions on how people conceive of their own reproductive interests.

In 1982, the French philosopher Michel Foucault outlined four technologies by which humans have come to understand themselves: technologies of production, of signs, of power, and of self. These technologies, he noted, "hardly ever function separately"; indeed, understanding how one technology might interact with another is crucial in understanding how there is very little knowledge we can accept at face value; what presents itself as a technology of production, like IVF, as "just" a medical intervention, is also a technology of late capitalism and pronatalism. "Perhaps," he wrote, "I've insisted too much on the technology of domination and power. I am more and more interested in the interaction between oneself and others and in the technologies of individual domination, the history of how an individual acts upon himself, in the technology of self." Foucault was well known for his studies of sexuality, mental illness, discipline, and punishment, and now he wanted to consider more closely how individuals attained "a certain state of happiness, purity, wisdom, perfection, or immortality" by way of "a certain number of operations on their own bodies and souls, thoughts, conduct, and way of being." The use of the word *operation* here seems revealing. Foucault is recasting self-improvement and/or self-knowledge as a series of surgical interventions, as procedures enacted on one's own life.

It is precisely in this sense that IVF has also been a technology of self in my own life. Many moons ago, long before the events of this book, a man I was dating sent me a link to a BBC article: scientists, it said, were looking for an adventurous woman to be a surrogate for the embryo of a cloned Neanderthal human being. He liked the language, he said: an "adventurous" woman. I read other scientists' reactions to the cloning proposal. Many predicted problems. Until then, there had only been one real attempt to clone an extinct animal: in 2003, scientists managed to clone a Pyrenean ibex, which went extinct in 2000. They were working with substantially better odds: unlike Neanderthals, they had a complete DNA sample to work with (rather than a partial one). Still, the numbers were remarkable: 439 ibex embryos were created, and of those, seven resulted in pregnancies. Only one ibex made it to birth, and it died a few minutes later, from lung defects. Commenting on the proposal to clone a Neanderthal human, one scientist noted that it would "require dozens of women, many of whom would almost certainly go through the trauma of miscarriage and stillbirths that appear to be inevitable when it comes to cloning." It would take a camp of adventurous women; a small city of them.

That night, I dreamed of it. I saw a Soviet-style city in the middle of the taiga, composed entirely of crumbling apartment buildings. On each balcony sat a pregnant woman, rocking in her chair, watching the sunset over hills that were so far away they seemed closer to thought than to earth. These women lived alone—one in each apartment—but they spoke to each other across the balcony walls about television, their doctors, each other. I could hear the beep of monitoring devices strapped to their bellies, the rattling castors of the machines they pushed along the corridors. I could hear cicadas in the fields beyond. They sat and looked and spoke with the patience of saints in old paintings, waiting to see if theirs was the egg that passed through the eye of the needle: if they would be the one to give birth to a healthy past. I would like to live in that city, I wrote in my notebook next morning. I would like to live alongside that grief and that courage. Their kitchens had hardly anything in them. There was a shelf, a few pots and pans, a bowl.

When I had this dream, I was years from finding out my FSH levels. I suppose I must've known about IVF, but only dimly. It is the only prophecy I have ever unknowingly written about my life. Now I see that I have always been drawn or fixed by images of groups of women, sitting, waiting: in a manor house, in a dusty clinic. IVF may reinforce existing conservative visions of the family, but it has also amplified very specific currents in my own life—has grafted, with barely any resistance, onto my preexisting technologies of self. Medicine did not scare me. I grew up shuttling between my mother's waiting room and my father's office next to a laboratory. I would like to say that IVF has served as an extension to my life, rather than an interruption of it, like one of Franklin's handblown pipettes, handled with skill. I would like to say that it has given me access to more freedom: and it has. Yet much of this was done under the cover of a conservative vision of a family, in viviparous days, when I was routinely mistaken for a wife.

The way *out* of this net, Franklin suggests, is through analogy. In *Biological Relatives*, she returns to that hatch: the architectural equivalent of a hyphen, pointing out the differences between our ways of characterizing and describing life in the IVF clinic (with its focus on the singularity of the embryo, its cellular enactment of a union), and how we understand the cultivation of stem-cell lines in colonies of "immortalized, regenerative, anonymized, and totipotent cells." Franklin points out the ways in which these two different thinking systems converge, like different bodies of water. What would change if we permitted ourselves to think of reproduction as the creation of a new cell line, as a set of potentialities rather than a singularity? What does it do to our understanding of cell duplication to think of human-centered models of growth rather than machine-centered ones? Analogies reflect ideological pressures, and changes in analogies and metaphors might harbor or foment paradigm shifts. This is not old news: Franklin invokes Marilyn Strathern's discussion of the "domaining effect," which is when ideas, by way of analogy, move from one cultural or social context to another. Analogies *pull* ideas in a certain direction. They cast the thought out, in a slightly longer arc, into a different body of water. The invitation often happens quietly, without fuss, but the underlying schema of attitudes and assumptions also shifts.

Susan Squier, in her wonderful study of visions of ectogenesis in nineteenth- and twentieth-century literature, writes that "analogies are neither merely artificial grafts, nor wholly innocent." Not coincidentally, Squier's analogy recalls Mitchison's graft—her child Ariel—who is an excellent example of the analogical impulse to reconceptualize reproduction. On the one hand, we recognize Mitchison's metonymy for pregnancy: when Mary is growing Ariel, who is attached to her thigh, her breasts swell and the areolae darken, her taste for food changes, and her thoughts turn inward, preoccupied with communicating with this creature. As the graft grows, Mary's movement is impeded, and she fashions a sling to carry her graft in. She tries to communicate with the creature by listening to music, concentrating on number theory, and looking at art, "both figurative and non-figurative art of various schools in the past and present." This line of thinking is not so far away from that of current mothers who play music to their child in utero, or who decide to focus on particular thought patterns; but by naming the knowledge systems rather than texts, and by removing any neotenous image of an infant, this scene renders, as a tableau, what it looks like to re-imagine gestation and gesture. When it is discovered that Ariel can communicate via number theory, pressing the spacewoman's palm with a tentacle in soft taps, it is heralded as a trans-species accomplishment. This is what it looks like to fully honor the difference of a being that grew from you. Nothing is taken for granted: all is curiosity. Squier points out that there is a distinct tradition running through English literature—from Charles Kingsley through Aldous and Julian Huxley, through J. B. S. Haldane and on to Naomi Mitchison—of imagining various displacements of reproduction. In other words, although the Warnock Report helped establish a "cultural education" about the embryo and new reproductive technologies in the 1980s in the United Kingdom, it is quite possible there are other voices and precedents that have made that hatch in Guy's Hospital more conceivable. Whereas only ten percent of couples with excess embryos in the United States decide to donate them to research, and though the United States and United Kingdom share many cultural attitudes toward families, *70 percent* of couples in the United Kingdom donate their excess embryos to research.

I had always thought my own ambivalence was a problem to solve. Now, I think it is a feature of reproductive capacity. There is no getting around or away from it. There is no *problem* with it. Ambivalence could be considered a constitutive component of biological relativity, the tension between the knowledge that while there is biological cause and effect, in a complex, multi-level system there is no privileged level of biology of causation. You could fall pregnant, and you might not fall pregnant. That hovering duality might not be something to suffer, or escape from. How much of a relief it would've been to remind myself earlier that my vacillation was biologically structural, not a function of my choice or freedom. Those two-week waits might have proceeded differently if I had reminded myself, much more forcefully, that my body's ambivalence was not something I could control. Yes, there were things I could probably do to help, but my will was not all-encompassing. This is not to disregard societal expectation, or a much longer history of racialized pronatalist coercion, but simply to recast what I saw as a failure to resolve, with imagination or resources, the way I was living. Indeed, it was only when my ambivalence was removed—resolved *for* me—that I panicked.

During the time I've taken to write this book, a number of my friends have experienced infertility. It's common knowledge what I chose to do, and that I have been writing about it, but some of them have not been able to talk to me because it is too painful to talk to a woman, even a friend, who has been successful, and who has a child. They cannot come to my house and see Anika's toys on the floor, her drawings on the walls: they need to be careful with what they allow to come close. I remember that feeling well. Their assessment of how and why they want children might be completely different from my own, but it is too painful to compare notes. Our grief makes us mute. The women in my dream spoke to each other; the women in my waiting rooms did not; and while the women online spoke to each other, I had no idea how to speak to them. I have spent a lot of time thinking about the stethoscope, about paper, rolled into a tube, how Western science translates sound into sight, and also about how writing propulsively reverses that current, moving from sight to the silent recreation of a voice. This is why there need to be more narrative accounts of women's reproductive frame of mind, more stories, on which analogies grow like polyps, seeding meaning of which even the writer may not be aware. If the stethoscope was part of a movement to standardize medical care, which also constructed a hierarchy of perception and shame (when to look, when not to look, how looking might be a transgression), then another piece of paper can also reorder these expectations. There just need to be many more of them.

Let me climb through that hatch, and find myself in a bedroom. In the corner is a wardrobe with the door open; inside, hanging on the back of the door, is a mirror. I can approach, and stand in front of the mirror, naked. It is late afternoon, and I can hear the wind in the trees outside. Here is my body. Here are my eyes, regarding me. I inspect my skin, my freckles, watching for sudden expansions or implosions. My mother is on her sixth melanoma. I look for her echo on my arms and legs. As my child grows, I have developed a completely different appreciation for cellular renewal, for the silent knitting together, the sloughing off. My periods still come, though they are shorter, the blood darker. My hair changes color. Grooves on my face deepen. I think of those pills in the chimney back in New Zealand yellowing and peeling; the chicken carcass on the bench, gangly with loose ends of flesh; my own intestines, how mysterious they seem to me. My own interior design. Pinkness and blueness and whiteness and redness and blackness, all of it slick and shuddering with my life, all the while waiting, all the while decaying. All that I can and cannot imagine. This is not an image, but a film: continuing until it doesn't.

The process of deciding to have a child has changed my phe-

nomenology of self: how I value an embryo or a child colors everything I do or see. How I think or perceive the world cannot be peeled
away from my reproductive experience. This knowledge is gendered, in the sense that I am easily identified as a woman by others,
but I find that my sense of reproduction reveals less about being a
woman than it does my own mortality as a human being raising
another. I wish I had known this was true before I had Anika, and
known that *not* having a child is just as much a reproductive experience as having one. I would've learned this with age, but I'm not sure
how long it would've taken; I was so single-minded for so long, and
I had constructed a life that allowed me to move, unimpeded, on a
straight course, never hitting my target. I'm not sure how my body
would've confronted me. Motherhood simply sped up the process.
Now I am multi-minded, a Scylla of attention and breath and thinking, so much more aware of the way my mind darts from this page
to the cry of children outside, aware of the way other people are also
multi-minded, branching: how difficult it is to fix anything still. I
think of von Baer's egg, that dot; my own cellular matter, a meteor
trail spread out through the world. I think of my two embryos, and
what life awaits them if they are passed through the hatch.

We were climbing stairs of a museum together the other day,
Anika holding my hand, when she pointed at a painting in front of
us and described it as a "self-portrait." I was astonished that she'd
picked up the word. Self-portraits are attempts to integrate an inner
vision and an outer recognizable reality, to create a reconciliation
between the body and mind. They are a technology of self. She understood the charge of the painting in front of us: that confrontation.
She looked at the painting's eyes, the man's mouth. She understood
why he wanted to paint, and she wanted to hurry home and do it

too. These days, Anika and I now sit in front of a mirror, paintbrush in hand, paper in front of us, and I pretend to paint but really watch her eyes move from herself to the page, watch the way her attention narrows, then branches. I marvel at the way she sets up a rhythm of perception for herself in the world. This is the looking that involves life.

One day when she was five, she painted more than thirty paintings in her notebook in quick succession, all of the same thing: a red boat on the sea. She refined the iconography, moving quickly: blue line, red curve, over and over again. Her determination to cover such ground amazed me. Her appetite for the symbolic is deepening, expanding at a speed I cannot track. She is creating her own hatches now. "I'm going to fill the *whole book up*," she said. And she did.

Acknowledgments

This book grew from an essay I published in *Tell You What: Great New Zealand Nonfiction 2016*, and I'm grateful to the book's editors, Susanna Andrew and Jolisa Gracewood, for their early support. My thanks go to *Avidly* and *Southwestern Review* for allowing me to publish very early work on other strands of this book's argument. McDowell gave me the time and space of a residency to develop the book proposal, which then developed with the stalwart support of Don Fehr, my agent at Trident Media Group. I am so lucky that I met Courtney Young at Riverhead Books. She has been patient, precise, and empathetic. Her team—including Jacqueline Shost and Annie Gottlieb—have been remarkable.

I'd like to thank the team at Bourn Hall for so graciously welcoming me, and for setting up interviews with staff and former patients. Willem Ombelet took time out of what was obviously a very busy day to speak at length with me about his work, and to give me a tour of his clinic. I'd also like to thank the women across the United States willing to speak with me about embryo donation and adoption. It is never comfortable to see another person's representation of you in print, and it should go without saying that these are my perceptions, with all the distortions of self and memory that come with it. For that reason, I also thank my parents and family for their forbearance: they raised me to take risks, and this one involves them.

ACKNOWLEDGMENTS

This book was written in the corners of days, in between working at NYU and caring for Anika. I want to thank and acknowledge the people who gave me more time to write. Bethany Godsoe fought for me to take a three-month leave. Shahzad was right to insist at Anika's birth that four hours of writing time was immediately possible, and he and Gyda have given me many more hours since, including the time to write these exact words. JoyAnn Chandler and Julia Easterlin looked after Anika before she went to daycare and gave her boundaries and Polish punk. A succession of marvelous teachers and school administrators at Brooklyn Free Space and Muse Academy minimized the disruption of the pandemic. This book has also hugely benefited from some wonderful readers: Sarra Alpert, C. Ray Borck, Megan Davidson, Doug Dibbern, Tania Friedel, Mary Kosut, Richard Larson, Beth Machlan, Lisa Jean Moore, Amira Pierce, and Stephanie Schiavenato. Their questions, advice, and support were crucial. Charles Gute provided invaluable fact-checking support.

Throughout these years, Zac has always righted my ship. The soundtrack to the writing of this book has been his voice in the living room, reading to Anika.

And to Anika: this is why Mum stares at the computer so much. I love you. Thank you for being such an amazing daughter.

Notes

1. GRAFT

5 **Aldous's brother, Julian Huxley, also wrote:** Both Julian and Aldous Huxley were raised on literature that described artificial wombs without naming them as such. The Victorian children's book *The Water-Babies: A Fairy Tale for a Land-Baby* (London: Macmillan, 1863) by Charles Kingsley—which the Huxleys read as children—specifically named their own grandfather, T. H. Huxley, the defender of Darwinism, as a man of science interested in putting a water baby in a bottle, and perhaps dissecting it. Both brothers were quick to make fiction sound like science, to cloak radical imagination in the tones of empirical observation. For discussions of Haldane, Mitchison, and Huxley (which include this reference to Kingsley), see Susan Merrill Squier's *Babies in Bottles: Twentieth-Century Visions of Reproductive Technology* (New Brunswick, NJ: Rutgers University Press, 1994).

5 **France was producing 60,000 children annually:** J. B. S. Haldane, "Daedalus, or, Science and the Future," a paper read to the Heretics, Cambridge, February 4, 1923, archived at https://www.marxists.org/archive/haldane/works/1920s/daedalus.htm.

7 **"Communication science is so essentially womanly":** Naomi Mitchison, *Memoirs of a Spacewoman* (London: Victor Gollancz, 1962; repr., Glasgow: Kennedy & Boyd, 2011), 17.

7 **"how much we are ourselves constructed bi-laterally":** Mitchison, *Memoirs of a Spacewoman*, 18.

8 **Right now, the odds:** These statistics are maddeningly hard to pin down. It depends on the clinic, country, age of the woman, etc. IVF clinics employ statistics for their quantitatively authoritative feel, but in retrospect, having gone through the experiences I have, as well as having researched this book, I would strongly recommend that they be taken with a very large grain of salt.

2. 14.3

14 **"Essentially, an elevated Day 3 FSH value":** "IVF Success Rates," Reproductive Medicine Associates of Michigan, accessed November 1, 2021, https:// www.rmami.com/about-success-rates-reproductive-medicine-of-michigan .html#:~:text=Essentially%2C%20an%20elevated%20Day%203,not %20favorably%20change%20this%20prognosis.

15 **Most health organizations:** It is worth noting how gendered this definition is. There is very little room for nonbinary and trans people here.

3. PAPER, SPOON, CYST

19 **Until the beginning of the twentieth century:** Yes, there is a distinct echo here with psychoanalysis, which also developed in the first half of the twentieth century.

20 **In 1760, the Austrian physician:** Malcolm Nicolson, "Examining the Body Since 1750," in *The Routledge History of Sex and the Body: 1500 to the Present*, ed. Sarah Toulalan and Kate Fisher (London: Routledge, 2013), 108.

21 **The heart's percussive sounds:** Nicolson, "Examining the Body Since 1750," 110.

21 **in Paris alone, by 1830:** H. K. Walker, "The Origins of the History and Physical Examination," in *Clinical Methods: The History, Physical, and Laboratory Examinations*, 3rd ed., ed. H. K. Walker, W. D. Hall, and J. W. Hurst (Boston: Butterworths, 1990), https://www.ncbi.nlm.nih.gov/books/NBK458/.

21 **"began a process by which the basis of the understanding":** Nicolson, "Examining the Body Since 1750," 111.

22 **virtually refused to be touched:** Nicolson, 91.

22 **"at your peril both as a practitioner":** Nicolson, 113.

22 **A follow-up photograph:** Nicolson, 112.

23 **"It is a profession for which I have the utmost contempt":** J. Marion Sims, *The Story of My Life* (New York: D. Appleton and Company, 1884), 116.

23 **"no clinical advantages":** Sims, *The Story of My Life*, 139.

24 **"trust entirely to nature than to . . . doctors":** Sims, 234.

26 **6 percent of the enslaved people:** Steven Mintz, "Historical Context: American Slavery in Comparative Perspective," The Gilder Lehrman Institute of American History, accessed November 1, 2021, https://www.gilderlehrman.org /history-resources/teaching-resource/historical-context-american-slavery -comparative-perspective.

26 **"Introducing the bent handle of the spoon":** Sims, *The Story of My Life*, 234–35.

27 **"Lucy's agony was extreme":** Sims, 238.

29 **"the dread of my young life":** Sims, 56.

30 **"which I cannot dwell upon":** John Brown, *Slave Life in Georgia: A Narrative of the Life, Sufferings, and Escape of John Brown, A Fugitive Slave* (London: W. M. Watts, 1855), 48.

30 **more generalized sense of moral outrage:** Harriet A. Washington, *Medical Apartheid: The Dark History of Medical Experimentation on Black Americans from Colonial Times to the Present* (New York: Doubleday, 2006).

34 **"A cyst produced echoes":** Ian Donald, "Apologia: How and Why Medical Sonar Developed," *Annals of the Royal College of Surgeons of England* 54, no. 3 (1974): 133.

34 **"plain or teat ended condoms":** Ian Donald, "Sonar: The Story of an Experiment," *Ultrasound in Medicine and Biology* 1, no. 2 (1974): 110.

35 **It was so difficult to determine:** For more information on the development of ultrasound technology, see Malcolm Nicolson and John E. E. Fleming, *Imaging and Imagining the Fetus: The Development of Obstetric Ultrasound* (Baltimore: Johns Hopkins University Press, 2013).

4. ALL MY POSTERITY

39 **"of all my posterity":** Elizabeth Appleton, quoted in Elaine Tyler May, *Barren in the Promised Land: Childless Americans and the Pursuit of Happiness* (New York: Basic Books / HarperCollins, 1995), 24.

40 **"probably without parallel in history":** Thomas Malthus, quoted in May, *Barren in the Promised Land*, 35.

40 **"to have an inordinate, and envious":** John Demos, quoted in May, 28.

41 **By the nineteenth century:** The average Anglo-colonial lifespan comes from Max Roser, Esteban Ortiz-Ospina, and Hannah Ritchie, "Life Expectancy," Our World in Data, last revised October 2019, https://ourworldindata.org /life-expectancy. The Native American figures come from Russell Thornton,

American Indian Holocaust and Survival: A Population History Since 1492 (Norman: University of Oklahoma Press, 1987).

41 **"There are regions in our own land":** Theodore Roosevelt, quoted in May, *Barren in the Promised Land*, 61.

41 **"race suicide among the rich":** May, 61.

41 **"The *patriotic* [my emphasis] enterprise":** George B. H. Swayze, quoted in May, 72.

42 **"Prevent young girls from":** May, 82.

42 **one of many efforts:** May, 64.

43 **We've come to think of the exponential increase:** The pill received FDA approval in 1960, but it wasn't until 1965 that the Supreme Court ruled that it could be advertised. By 1965, 1 out of 4 married women in the United States had taken the pill. "The Birth Control Pill: A History," Planned Parenthood, updated June 2015, https://www.plannedparenthood.org/files/1514/3518/7100/Pill_History_FactSheet.pdf.

44 **the average married couple:** Statistics on abortion rates and family sizes in nineteenth-century America are provided by May, *Barren in the Promised Land*, 44.

44 **1 abortion for every 6 live births:** May, 47.

44 **In 1878, the Michigan Board of Health:** May, 47.

45 **"abortion was a criminal offense":** May, 48.

45 **In 1911, a woman wrote:** May, 82–83.

45 **By the mid-1920s, the birth rate:** This statistic is contested by other studies that estimate the birth rate at around 3; as many statisticians note, record keeping is and was not what it should've been. It should be noted that there have frequently been statistically meaningful differences in birth rate by race across the United States.

46 **"We have discussed its possibilities":** "Anonymous, New York City," quoted in May, *Barren in the Promised Land*, 85–86.

47 **"I am forty years old":** Margaret Sanger, *Motherhood in Bondage* (Columbus: Ohio State University Press, 2000), 50.

47 **My aunt, a graphic designer:** Claire Patterson and Lindsay Quilter, *It's OK to Be You!: A Frank and Funny Guide to Growing Up* (Auckland: Tricycle Press, 1988).

50 **"most parents in human history":** Anna Rotkirch, "Baby Fever and Longing for Children," in *Fertility Rates and Population Decline: No Time for Children?*, ed. Ann Buchanan and A. Rotkirch (London: Palgrave Macmillan, 2013), 252.

51 **In different countries, women:** Rotkirch, "Baby Fever and Longing for Children," 249.

51 **Probably 12 percent of:** May, *Barren in the Promised Land,* 289.

53 **"Is the patient a cold":** Elaine Tyler May, "Nonmothers as Bad Mothers: Infertility and the 'Maternal Instinct,'" in *Bad Mothers: The Politics of Blame in Twentieth-Century America,* ed. Molly Ladd-Taylor and Lauri Umansky (New York: New York University Press, 1998), 204.

5. SEEING

61 **Sperm were first seen:** See https://lensonleeuwenhoek.net for an exhaustive general account of Leeuwenhoek's life.

61 **"They were furnished with a thin tail":** Leeuwenhoek's letters have been archived (in Dutch and English) by The Digital Library for Dutch Literature (DBNL). The description of sperm is in letter no. 35, November 1677, https://www.dbnl.org/tekst/leeu027alle02_01/leeu027alle02_01_0015.php#b0035\.

62 **albeit with some reserve:** For more detail about Henry Oldenburg's resistance to publishing or announcing some of Leeuwenhoek's findings, see Nick Lane, "The Unseen World: Reflections on Leeuwenhoek (1677) 'Concerning Little Animals,'" *The Royal Society* 370, no. 1666 (April 19, 2015): 20140344, https://doi.org/10.1098/rstb.2014.0344.

64 **"minuscule and well-developed":** Karl Ernst von Baer, "On the Genesis of the Ovum of Mammals and of Man," trans. Charles Donald O'Malley, *Isis* 47, no. 2 (June 1956): 120.

67 **is hardly the only way:** I am indebted to Jane Maienschein's *Embryos Under the Microscope: The Diverging Meanings of Life* (Cambridge, MA: Harvard University Press, 2014) for her work on the ways in which a Western modern scientific tradition has visualized embryos.

68 **"sucking its thumb":** Geraldine Lux Flanagan, *The First Nine Months of Life* (New York: Simon & Schuster, 1962, 1982), 44, 50, 52, 54.

69 **"the back muscles contract":** Flanagan, *The First Nine Months of Life,* 44–45.

69 **"gain from these pages":** George W. Corner, foreword, in Flanagan, 7.

70 **"multitudinous vascular channels":** E. C. Amoroso and G. W. Corner, "Herbert McLean Evans, 1882–1971," *Biographical Memoirs of Fellows of the Royal Society* 18 (November 1972): 98, http://www.jstor.org/stable/769658\.

71 **From the 1970s on, a wave:** I am indebted to Rayna Rapp and Faye Ginsburg for their work on testing procedures and women's perception of their

reproductive abilities, in particular Rayna Rapp, *Testing Women, Testing the Fetus: The Social Impact of Amniocentesis in America* (New York: Routledge, 2000); Faye D. Ginsburg, *Contested Lives: The Abortion Debate in an American Community* (Berkeley and Los Angeles: University of California Press, 1989); Barbara Katz Rothman, *The Tentative Pregnancy: How Amniocentesis Changes the Experience of Motherhood* (New York: W. W. Norton & Company, 1986, 1993); and Tine M. Gammeltoft, *Haunting Images: A Cultural Account of Selective Reproduction in Vietnam* (Berkeley and Los Angeles: University of California Press, 2014).

71 **In her landmark study:** Lisa M. Mitchell, *Baby's First Picture: Ultrasound and the Politics of Fetal Subjects* (Toronto: University of Toronto Press, 2001).

6. HE SAID/HE SAID

75 **"to deliver a healthy baby":** Robert Edwards and Patrick Steptoe, *A Matter of Life: The Story of a Medical Breakthrough* (New York: William Morrow, 1980), 65.

76 **"The involvement of her facial":** Edwards and Steptoe, *A Matter of Life*, 65.

76 **"I had never seen women":** Edwards and Steptoe, 66.

77 **"competitive second son":** Robert Edwards, quoted in Daniel M. Davis, *The Secret Body: How the New Science of the Human Body Is Changing the Way We Live* (Princeton, NJ: Princeton University Press, 2021), 43.

79 **"Most of them I just poached":** Landrum Brewer Shettles, quoted in Mary Dodge and Gilbert Geis, *Stealing Dreams: A Fertility Clinic Scandal* (Boston: Northeastern University Press, 2003), 92.

80 **"the issues of fertilization":** Edwards and Steptoe, *A Matter of Life*, 48.

84 **"visible and crimson":** Aldous Huxley, *Brave New World* (London: Chatto & Windus, 1932), https://www.huxley.net/bnw/one.html.

84 **"Oh no, I *don't* want to play":** Huxley, *Brave New World*, https://www.huxley.net/bnw/one.html.

85 **"Ultimately we could have"** William Breckon, quoted in Andrea L. Bonnicksen, *In Vitro Fertilization: Building Policy from Laboratories to Legislatures* (New York: Columbia University Press, 1989), 14.

85 **"Doctors Start Baby Outside":** These headlines are quoted by Edwards and Steptoe, *A Matter of Life*, 100.

86 **"Something is happening":** Edwards and Steptoe, 93.

86 **"It was an unbelievable sight":** Edwards and Steptoe, 94.

87 "the innate capacity to": Edwards and Steptoe, 102.

88 They were there because their doctor: For a very detailed account of Landrum Shettles and Doris Del-Zio's attempt to fall pregnant, see Robin Marantz Henig's *Pandora's Baby: How the First Test Tube Babies Sparked the Reproductive Revolution* (Boston: Houghton Mifflin, 2004). She also offers accounts of Daniele Petrucci and *In His Image*.

88 "resembled a frothy chocolate": Henig, *Pandora's Baby*, 23.

99 "She was quietly determined": Edwards and Steptoe, *A Matter of Life*, 143.

101 "cell to cell along": Jamshed R. Tata, "One Hundred Years of Hormones," *EMBO Reports* 6, no. 6 (June 2005): 490–96.

101 In the 1920s, the American scientist: Edgar Allen, J. Wilbur Whitsett, and John W. Hardy, "The Follicular Hormone of the Hen Ovary," *Proceedings of the Society for Experimental Biology and Medicine* 21, no. 8 (May 1924): 500–503. As can be seen in this paper, Allen experimented on hens, rats, cows, guinea pigs, rabbits, and monkeys, and also tried injecting the extract into humans.

102 By the mid-1980s, demand outstripped: For information on Donini see Oliver Staley, "The Strange Story of a Fertility Drug Made with the Pope's Blessing and Gallons of Nun Urine," *Quartz*, June 26, 2016, https://qz.com/710516/the-strange-story-of-a-fertility-drug-made-with-the-popes-blessing-and-gallons-of-nun-urine/.

106 There is a story by: Hans Christian Andersen, "Thumbelina" or "Little Tiny" (1835), http://hca.gilead.org.il/li_tiny.html#:~:text=(1835),managed%2C%E2%80%9D%20said%20the%20fairy.

108 This first wave of feminist scholarship: Charis Thompson, *Making Parents: The Ontological Choreography of Reproductive Technologies* (Cambridge, MA: MIT Press, 2005).

109 "We established a vertical": Gena Corea, *The Mother Machine: Reproductive Technologies from Artificial Insemination to Artificial Wombs* (London: The Women's Press, 1988), 61.

110 "one of the oldest forms": Corea, *The Mother Machine*, 60.

110 partially inspired in their reproductive research: Corea, 136.

111 "in a society in which men": Corea, 3.

111 "may well be a demand": It's worth quoting Corea in full: "Since we live in a society where white people are valued more highly than those of color, these technologies will not affect all women equally. There will be no great

demand for the eggs of a black woman. But there may well be a demand for her womb—a womb which could gestate the embryo of a white woman and man." Corea, 2.

111 **"interests of the patriarchy":** Corea, 2.

111 **"Just as the patriarchal state":** Corea, 2.

112 **"fetus in utero has become":** Barbara Katz Rothman, *The Tentative Pregnancy: How Amniocentesis Changes the Experience of Motherhood* (New York: W. W. Norton & Company, 1986, 1993), 114.

113 **"enabling technology":** Marilyn Strathern, *After Nature: English Kinship in the Late Twentieth Century* (Cambridge: Cambridge University Press, 1992), 49.

114 **"Baby's face was looking":** Edwards and Steptoe, *A Matter of Life*, 178.

115 **one of Louise's earliest memories:** Louise Brown, *My Life as the World's First Test-Tube Baby* (Bristol: Bristol Books, 2015), 107.

117 **"Why should a lorry driver":** Louise Brown, *My Life as the World's First Test-Tube Baby*, 91.

7. WOMB WITH A VIEW

120 **designed a learning module:** You can see Colin Quilter's modeling embryology project referred to and archived here: https://thenode.biologists.com/teaching-embryology-to-undergraduates/photo/.

120 **"transcendently estimable" men:** Gena Corea, *The Mother Machine: Reproductive Technologies from Artificial Insemination to Artificial Wombs* (London: The Women's Press, 1988), 21.

120 **"the innate quality of such men":** Corea, *The Mother Machine*, 22.

121 **"These are top scientists":** Corea, 30.

123 **paternity is an "abstract idea":** Corea, summarizing Mary O'Brien's *The Politics of Reproduction* (1981) in *The Mother Machine*, 287.

123 **"can be broken down":** These binaries are quoted from FINRRAGE's "Declaration of Comilla," Kotbari, Comilla, Bangladesh, 1989, http://www.finrrage.org/wp-content/uploads/2016/03/FINRRAGE.pdf.

124 **statistically speaking, 50 percent:** Again, a statistic that is easy to generally accept but difficult to argue is highly accurate. For example, see "Women's Eggs and Age: The Genetics of Oocyte Ovarian Aging," from Shady Grove Fertility, accessed November 1, 2021, https://www.shadygrovefertility.com/article/how-does-age-impact-egg-supply/.

127 **lived experience of people:** Sarah Franklin's *Biological Relatives: IVF, Stem Cells, and the Future of Kinship* (Durham, NC: Duke University Press, 2013) offers an excellent overview of the first and second phases of feminist scholarship about reproductive technologies.

128 **"I just had a better feeling about it":** Charis Thompson, *Making Parents: The Ontological Choreography of Reproductive Technologies* (Cambridge, MA: MIT Press, 2005), 190.

129 **"The patients do not so":** Thompson, *Making Parents*, 191.

132 **"not narrated as a journey":** Franklin, *Biological Relatives*, 253.

133 **"character evolved in contact":** Ian Hacking, "Our Neo-Cartesian Bodies in Parts," *Critical Inquiry* 34, no. 1 (Autumn 2007): 81.

133 **"We regard our bodies as":** Hacking, "Our Neo-Cartesian Bodies in Parts," 83.

134 **"extract the typical from the storehouse":** Lorraine Daston and Peter Galison, *Objectivity* (New York: Zone Books, 2007), 58.

135 **"ideal splash—an Auto-Splash":** Daston and Galison, *Objectivity*, 13.

8. WORKING GIRL

144 **He measured, for instance:** Pierre Bourdieu's qualities of a home preferred by different social groupings are rendered in remarkable bar graphs in his 1979 book *Distinction: A Social Critique of the Judgment of Taste*, trans. Richard Nice (Cambridge, MA: Harvard University Press, 1984), 248.

145 **"the nation's tech-savvy singles":** Claritas's descriptions of these segments—their "segment narratives"—shift ever so slightly with each new report. Nonetheless, these quotes remain 90% accurate from year to year. For instance, see their 2020 version at https://environicsanalytics.com/docs/default-source /us---data-product-support-documents/claritas-prizm-premier-segment -narratives-ea.pdf.

149 **"a kind of general, enthusiastic commitment":** Roland Barthes, *Camera Lucida* (New York: Hill and Wang, 1980), 26–27.

151 **"somewhat unpleasant, though now":** J. B. S. Haldane, "Daedalus, or, Science and the Future," https://www.marxists.org/archive/haldane/works/1920s/dae dalus.htm.

9. AT NORTH FARM

158 **"Somewhere someone is traveling":** John Ashbery, "At North Farm," *A Wave* (New York: Viking Penguin, 1984), 1.

10. THE WALKING EGG

169 **Bourn Hall was barely:** The background of Bourn Hall has been compiled from multiple sources: Bourn Hall's website, in-person interviews with multiple staff members including Vivien Collins, Mike Macnamee, and Adam Burnley in October 2016, a phone interview with Ann Hartley (who was a patient there in 1981), and an in-person interview with Kay Elder in October 2016 (who has also published histories like this: https://blog.sciencemuseum.org.uk/bourn-hall-the-first-ivf-clinic/ in which she details the *Daily Mail*'s initial interest, opening patient numbers, etc.). Details about the property tend to be repeated in accounts of the early days of Bourn Hall, but stories about patients (the foreign wives of businessmen, and the "woman from Scarborough") were disclosed through in-person interviews with Bourn Hall staff.

172 **There were foreign wives:** Interview with Vivien Collins, who was formerly employed at Bourn Hall. Current staff are not aware of this situation, and believe Ms. Collins was trying to convey how new the treatment was, not any mistreatment of women.

176 **Patients would then have the flexibility:** All details about the founding and development of the Joneses' clinic are from Howard R. Jones, *In Vitro Fertilization Comes to America: Memoir of a Medical Breakthrough* (Williamsburg, VA: Jamestowne Bookworks, 2014).

177 **By 1984, there were clinics:** Michael Mulkay, *The Embryo Research Debate: Science and the Politics of Reproduction* (Cambridge: Cambridge University Press, 1997).

178 **From the 1970s onward:** Stephen S. Hall, *Merchants of Immortality: Chasing the Dream of Human Life Extension* (New York: Houghton Mifflin, 2003).

179 **"steady and general point":** Warnock Report available at https://www.hfea.gov.uk/media/2608/warnock-report-of-the-committee-of-inquiry-into-human-fertilisation-and-embryology-1984.pdf.

183 **definitions a "cultural education":** Marilyn Strathern's two 1992 publications, *After Nature: English Kinship in the Late 20th Century* (Cambridge: Cambridge University Press, 1992), and *Reproducing the Future: Essays on Anthropology, Kinship, and the New Reproductive Technologies* (Manchester, UK: Manchester University Press, 1992), are crucial to kinship studies.

185 **It was not surprising that:** For an account of risks taken by American clinics offering in vitro fertilization in the 1980s and 1990s, see Liza Mundy, *Everything Conceivable: How the Science of Assisted Reproduction Is Changing Men, Women, and the World* (New York: Alfred A. Knopf, 2007; paperback: Anchor Books, 2007).

187   who moved in 1987: Willem Ombelet, author's interview, October 2016.

187   In Africa, the percentage: I relied in particular on the following two articles
      in summarizing attitudes toward infertility in Africa: Marcia C. Inhorn and
      Pasquale Patrizio, "Infertility around the Globe: New Thinking on Gender, Re-
      productive Technologies and Global Movements in the 21st Century," *Human
      Reproduction Update* 21, no. 4 (July–August 2015): 411–26; and Willem Ombe-
      let, Ian Cooke, Silke Dyer, Gamal Serour, and Paul Devroey, "Infertility and the
      Provision of Infertility Medical Services in Developing Countries," *Human Re-
      production Update* 14, no. 6 (November–December 2008): 605–21.

187   In 2001, at a WHO meeting: Abdallah S. Daar and Zara Merali, "Infertility
      and Social Suffering: The Case of ART in Developing Countries," in *Current
      Practices and Controversies in Assisted Reproduction*, ed. E. Vayena, P. J. Rowe, and
      P. D. Griffin (Geneva: World Health Organization, 2002), 15–21.

188   Nonetheless, a 2004 study: Shea O. Rutstein and Iqbal H. Shah, *Infecundity,
      Infertility, and Childlessness in Developing Countries*, Demographic and Health Sur-
      veys (DHS) Comparative Reports 9 (Calverton, MD: ORC Macro and World
      Health Organization, 2004).

189   There has always been some variation: For accounts of IVF tourism, see *Fer-
      tility Holidays: IVF Tourism and the Reproduction of Whiteness* by Amy Speier (New
      York: New York University Press, 2016). Speier focuses on the Czech Republic.
      For other reproductive inequities to do with surrogacy, see Amrita Pande,
      Wombs in Labor: Transnational Commercial Surrogacy in India (New York: Columbia
      University Press, 2014).

189   Though the Congo's birth rate: Mortality, birth, and infertility rates in the Re-
      public of Congo and Belgium are calculated from www.Statista.com, accessed
      November 1, 2021.

192   If you could find a clinician: The price changes in various articles; some list it
      as $250, others as $750. This is usually a function of fluctuating currency and
      costs of materials.

11. LOOK! LOOK!

205   "As child is equivalent with imagination": James Hillman, "The Bad Mother:
      An Archetypal Approach," in *Fathers and Mothers: Five Papers on the Archetypal
      Background of Family Psychology*, ed. Patricia Berry (Zürich: Spring Publications,
      1973). This exact set of sentences has infuriated other writing mothers: it's also
      quoted by Rachel Cusk in her book *A Life's Work* (London: Picador, 2001).

205 **When Anika was barely:** Peter Linenthal, *Look Look!* (New York: Dutton Books for Young Readers, 1998).

12. SNOWFLAKE

218 **At its height in 1970:** Exact numbers are difficult to confirm, but there is consensus that 1970 was probably the height of adoptive practices in the United States. See annual reports from the Child Welfare Information Gateway, part of the US Department of Health and Human Services. For an overview of international adoption markets, see Kathryn Joyce's *The Child Catchers: Rescue, Trafficking, and the New Gospel of Adoption* (New York: PublicAffairs, 2013), and Jane Jeong Trenka, Julia Chinyere Oparah, and Sun Yung Shin, *Outsiders Within: Writing on Transracial Adoption* (Boston: South End Press, 2006).

218 **in a country where the average:** In Ghana, for example, the minimum wage is $482 USD a month as of 2018. It should be noted here that $5,000 is more accurately the price paid to the biological parent for a child, and that the cost to the adoptive parent (including application and adoption fees and permits, etc.) is closer to between $20,000 and $40,000 USD.

219 **"physical, emotional, psychological, and spiritual":** Nancy Newton Verrier, *The Primal Wound: Understanding the Adopted Child* (Baltimore: Gateway Press, 1993), xvi. For an extraordinary account of this trauma for women who gave up infants, see Ann Fessler, *The Girls Who Went Away: The Hidden History of Women Who Surrendered Children for Adoption in the Decades before Roe v. Wade* (New York: Penguin Press, 2006).

220 **In 1997, Ron Stoddart:** This narrative is reconstructed by Stephen S. Hall in *Merchants of Immortality: Chasing the Dream of Human Life Extension* (New York: Houghton Mifflin, 2003).

221 **"She cried for 2 months":** Doug and Valarie Grindle, "Our Embryo Adoption Story," Nightlight Christian Adoptions, accessed November 1, 2021, https://nightlight.org/2009/06/our-embryo-adoption-story/.

223 **By 1944, the collection:** For accounts of Wilhelm His and Franklin Mall, see Lynn Morgan, *Icons of Life: A Cultural History of Human Embryos* (Berkeley and Los Angeles: University of California Press, 2009).

223 **"we owe to your kindness":** Morgan, *Icons of Life*, 75.

223 **"taken from the uterus":** Morgan, 136.

224 **"increasingly distressed to think":** Morgan, 107.

225 **Some studies estimate the percentage:** For example, see Christopher R. Newton, Ann McDermid, Francis Tekpetey, and Ian S. Tummon, "Embryo Donation: Attitudes toward Donation Procedures and Factors Predicting Willingness to Donate," *Human Reproduction* 18, no. 4 (April 2003): 878–84, https://doi.org/10.1093/humrep/deg169.

225 **I spoke to ten women:** This was a highly unscientific or sociologically unmethodological study; the women were recommended to me through my contacts with embryo adoption agencies. Their reticence seemed even more interesting to me given that these people were all naturally pro–embryo adoption.

231 **It's now the case:** The Virtual Human Embryo Project: https://www.ehd.org/virtual-human-embryo/.

13. THROUGH THE HATCH

242 **"when to cut them":** Sarah Franklin, *Biological Relatives: IVF, Stem Cells, and the Future of Kinship* (Durham, NC: Duke University Press, 2013), 84.

242 **"Even in this ultramodern":** Franklin, *Biological Relatives*, 83.

242 **"inhabit each other's space":** Franklin, 78.

243 **"Embryos are like photograph film":** Aldous Huxley, *Brave New World* (London: Chatto & Windus, 1932), https://www.huxley.net/bnw/one.html.

243 **His laboratory—and many others:** For more information on William Harvey, read Thomas Wright's *William Harvey: A Life in Circulation* (Oxford, UK: Oxford University Press, 2012).

245 **bowls of hot soup:** Franklin's analogy. Franklin, *Biological Relatives*, 79.

246 **"As Foucault might have":** Franklin, 6.

246 **"a degree of flexibility":** Franklin, 6–7.

246 **"believe you will succeed":** Franklin, 7.

247 **"form of social existence":** Donna Haraway, quoted in Franklin, *Biological Relatives*, 71–72.

248 **"within heterosexual, wealthy contexts":** Haraway, "The Ironic Dream of a Common Language for Women in the Integrated Circuit: Science, Technology, and Socialist Feminism in the 1980s or A Socialist Feminist Manifesto for Cyborgs," 1983, https://dimitris.apeiro.gr/files/papers/Bodies/Haraway_The_Ironic_Dream.htm.

249 **"I know no better stance":** Haraway paraphrased by Franklin, 71.

249 **"strange folding":** Franklin, *Biological Relatives*, 7.

250 **"hardly ever function separately":** Michel Foucault, *Technologies of the Self: A Seminar with Michel Foucault*, ed. Luther H. Martin, Huck Gutman, and Patrick H. Hutton (Amherst: University of Massachusetts Press, 1988), 18.

250 **"I've insisted too much":** Foucault, *Technologies of the Self*, 18–19.

251 **an adventurous woman:** The phrase "adventurous woman" appeared to originate from an interview Professor George Church gave the German magazine *Der Spiegel* (published January 15, 2013), which was then translated and published in multiple English-speaking news outlets around the world. https://www.spiegel.de/wissenschaft/medizin/genforscher-george-church-will-neandertaler-klonen-a-877554.html. Church immediately challenged this reporting, suggesting the news outlets had mistranslated his words, but "an adventurous female human being" is a literal translation of the German original.

251 **"require dozens of women":** Alex Knapp, "Is It Possible to Clone A Neanderthal?" *Forbes*, January 20, 2013, https://www.forbes.com/sites/alexknapp/2013/01/20/is-it-possible-to-clone-a-neanderthal/?sh=68892a0666c4.

252 **"immortalized, regenerative, anonymized":** Franklin, *Biological Relatives*, 70.

253 **"analogies are neither merely":** Susan Merrill Squier, *Babies in Bottles: Twentieth-Century Visions of Reproductive Technology* (New Brunswick, NJ: Rutgers University Press, 1994), 25.

253 **"both figurative and non-figurative art":** Naomi Mitchison, *Memoirs of a Spacewoman* (London: Victor Gollancz, 1962; repr., Glasgow: Kennedy & Boyd, 2011), 50.